10-MINUTE AM/PM YOGA

Words and yoga instruction Eve Boggenpoel
Photography Adrian Volcinschi
Hair & make-up Danielle Hudson @ Artistic Licence
Clothes (cover) noballs Bamboo Strappy Bra, £36 (noballs.co.uk); ILU Supersoft Yoga Leggings, £39.99 (ilufitwear.com)
Clothes (inside) from a selection at ILU and noballs
Model Emily Eaton @ WModels
Props Yogamatters (yogamatters.com)

Editor Mary Comber
Art editor Holly Hall
Chief sub-editor Sheila Reid

Publisher Steven O'Hara
Publishing Director Dan Savage
Marketing Manager Charlotte Park
Commercial Director Nigel Hole

Printed by William Gibbons and Sons, Wolverhampton
ISBN 9781911639480

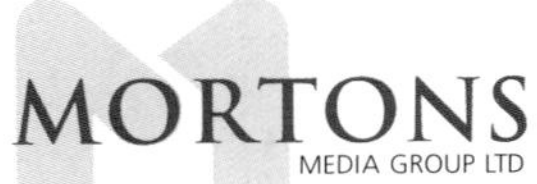

Published by Mortons Media Group Ltd,
Media Centre, Morton Way,
Horncastle, LN9 6JR
01507 529529

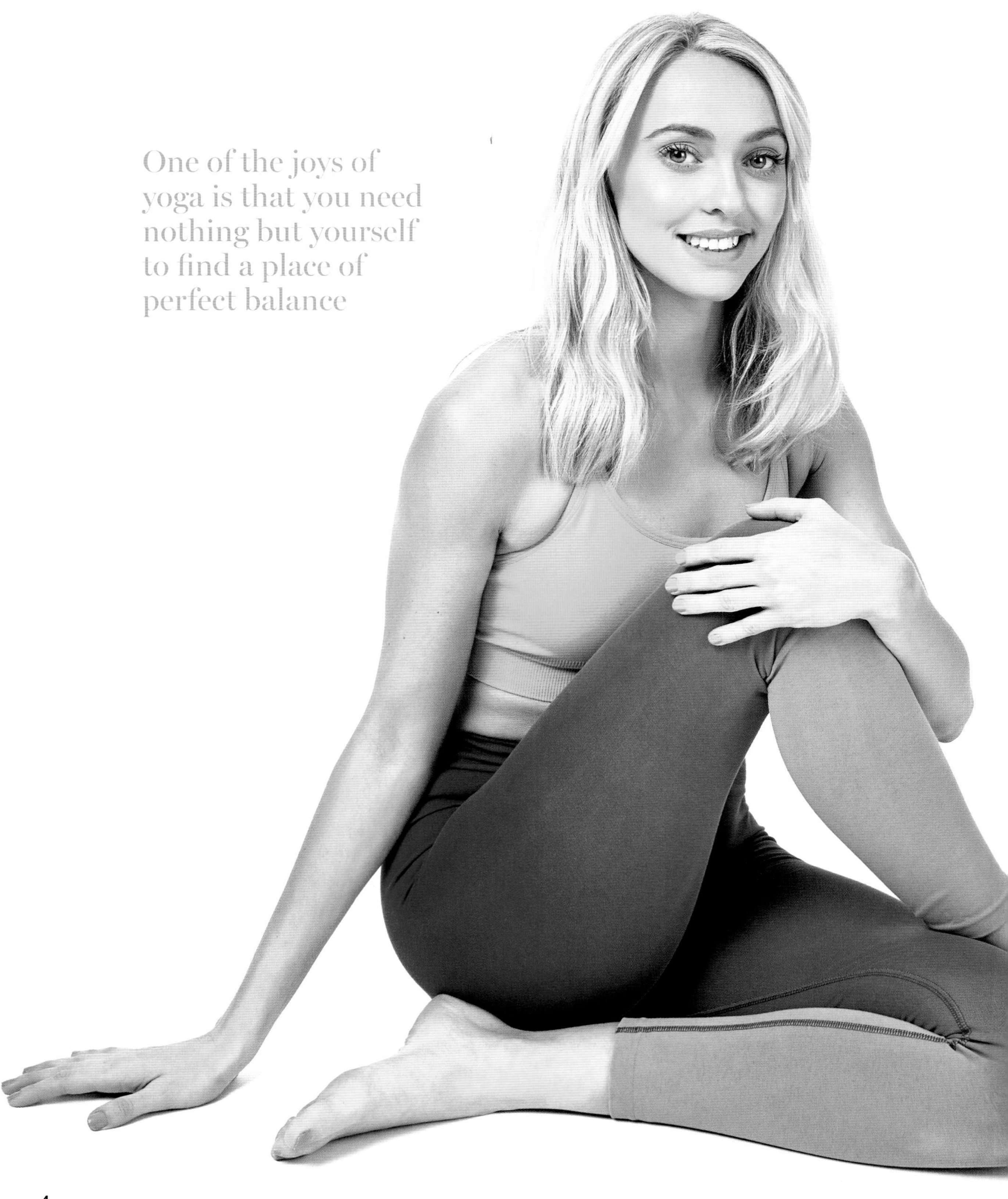

One of the joys of yoga is that you need nothing but yourself to find a place of perfect balance

Contents

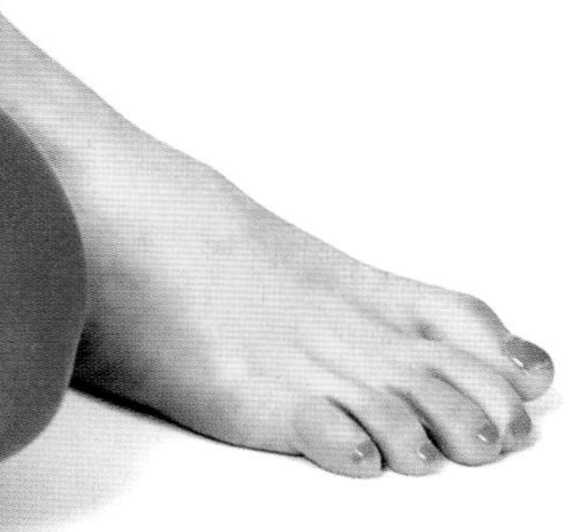

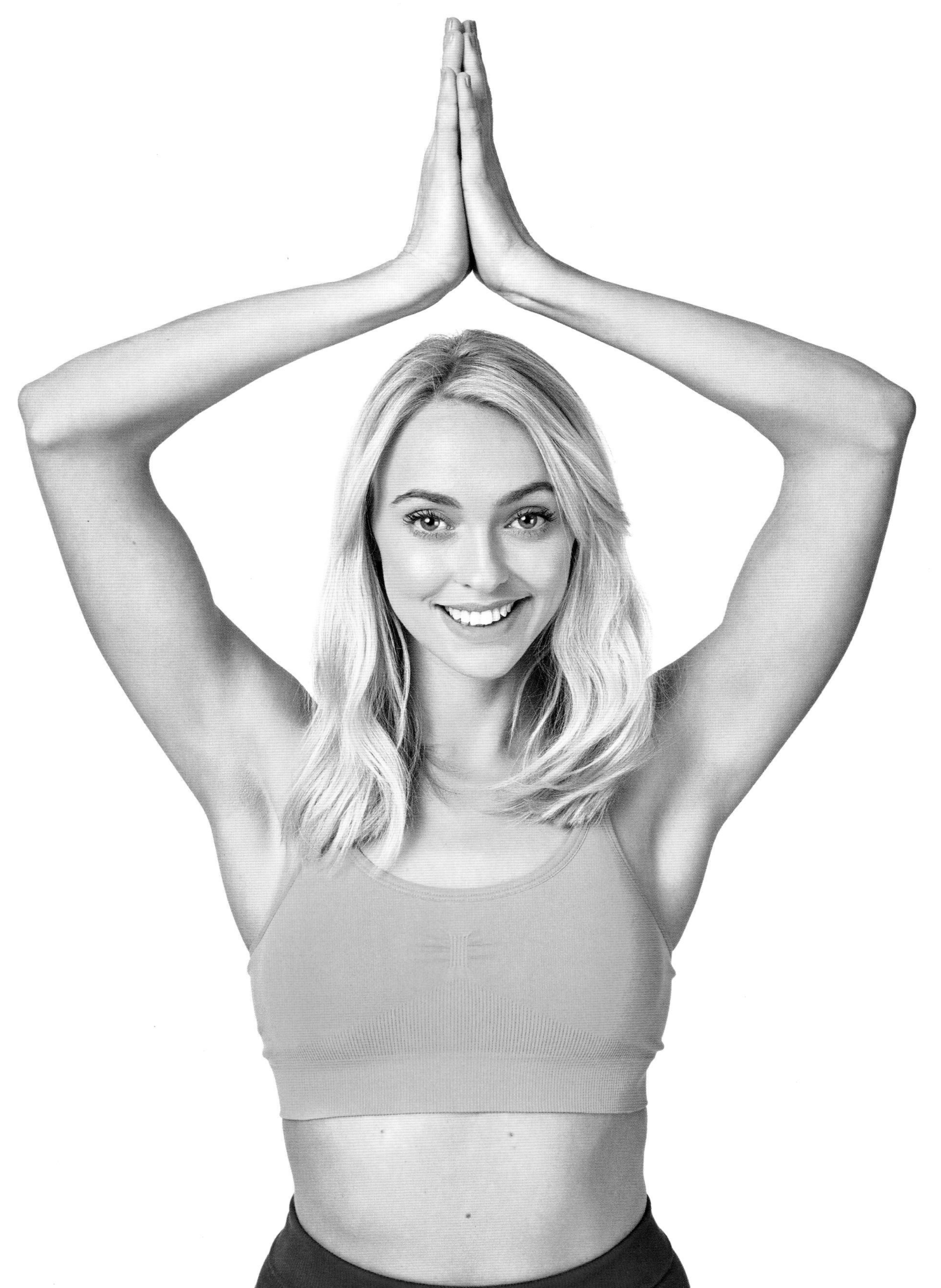

Welcome

There's nothing like the feeling of being in harmony with yourself and your surroundings. Some people find peace walking on a beach at sunset, while others are happiest when taking part in a tough sporting challenge.

One of the joys of yoga is that you need nothing but yourself to find a place of perfect balance. In *10-Minute AM/PM Yoga*, we've created a set of practices that will enhance your health and wellbeing, no matter where you are or what else is happening in your life.

Following an introduction to the basics of yoga, you'll find a carefully curated set of yoga practices to start and end your day. Turn to the energy-boosting morning sequences to find ways to supercharge your day, enhance your focus and boost concentration, then settle down with the restorative sequences and meditations in the evening to deeply relax and enjoy a better night's sleep.

You'll also find all the resources you need to practise yoga safely and get the most from your practice. Along the way, we hope you'll get to know yourself a little better and learn to be kind to yourself.

Eve

Eve Boggenpoel,
Author, *10-Minute AM/PM Yoga*

ABOUT THE AUTHOR

Eve Boggenpoel has been practising yoga and meditation for 25 years. Self-taught initially, her formal yoga journey began with a German Iyengar teacher when she learned to value the significance of good alignment, and went on to include Vinyasa and Yin styles with inspirational teachers Shiva Rea, Sarah Powers and Simon Low.

Eve is a qualified homeopath and health journalist, and author of several books, including *Yoga Calm*, *Mindfulness* and *Yoga Cures*. In *10-Minute AM/PM Yoga*, Eve brings together her in-depth knowledge of yoga, meditation and the Chinese practise of Qi gong to create an easy-to-use guide to enhance your wellbeing in everyday life.

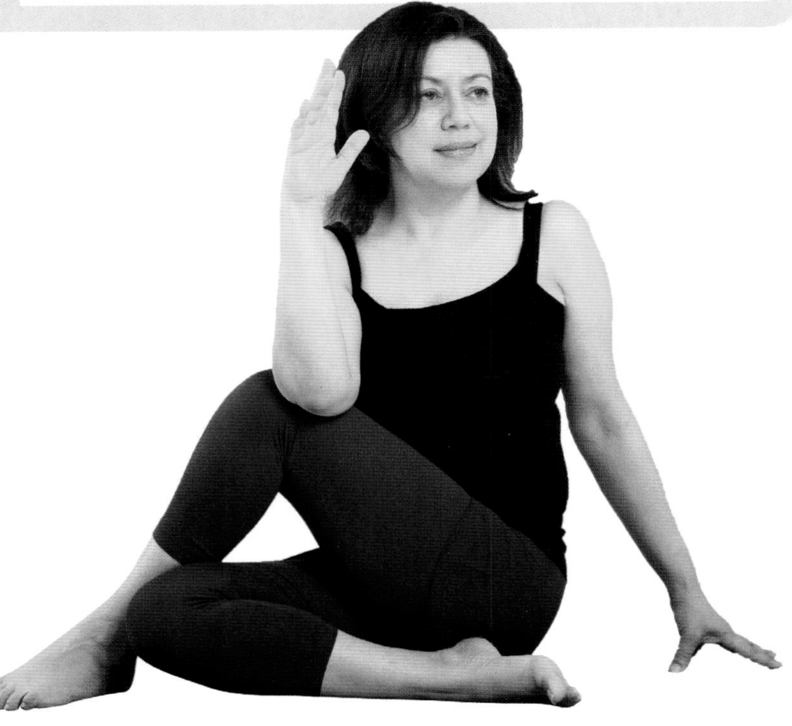

HOW TO USE THIS BOOK

Ready to start? Read these guidelines first to get maximum benefits from *10-Minute AM/PM Yoga*

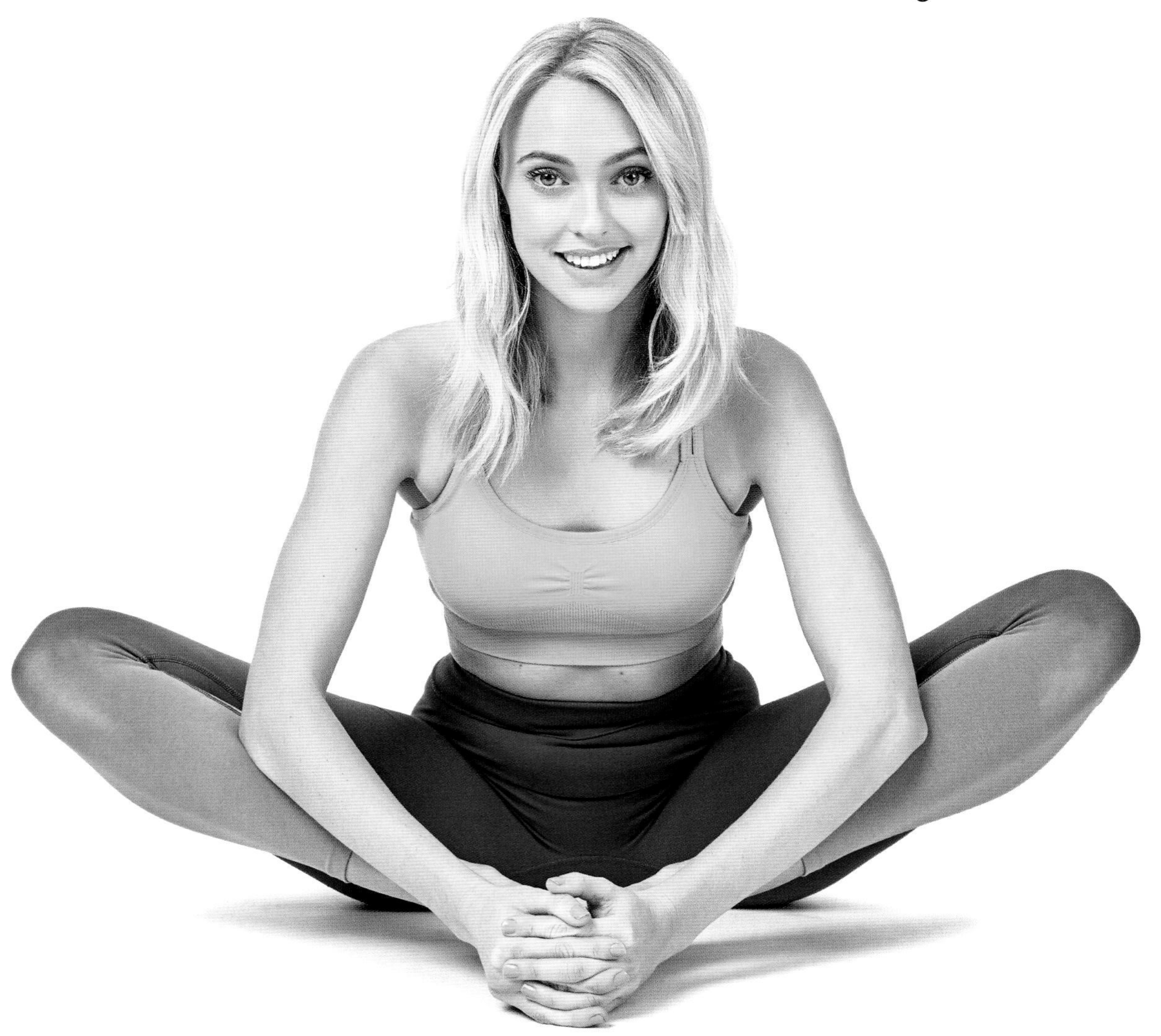

To get the most out of the sequences in this book it's important to learn the basics. Patience at the beginning will result in a safer, more effective practice – with more therapeutic benefits.

Start by trying the AM warm-up poses (p80) reading each pose carefully before attempting it. Listen to your body and feel how the poses (asanas) are stretching and loosening your muscles and joints.

Then move on to the AM postures (p22), starting with the standing poses. They form the basis of many other asanas, and the alignment techniques you are learning here will be repeated time and time again, so it's worth learning them well.

If you have limited time and want to start on one of the sequences (p78), note which poses are used in the sequence of your choice, for example AM stretch (p92), and focus on learning those, along with the relevant warm-up poses.

When you know how it feels to have balanced alignment in the AM poses, use this understanding in the PM poses (p60) and sequences (p102), allowing your body to sink more deeply into the poses for maximum relaxation benefits.

As always, trust your body and let it tell you what it needs.

Patience at the beginning will result in a safer, more effective practice

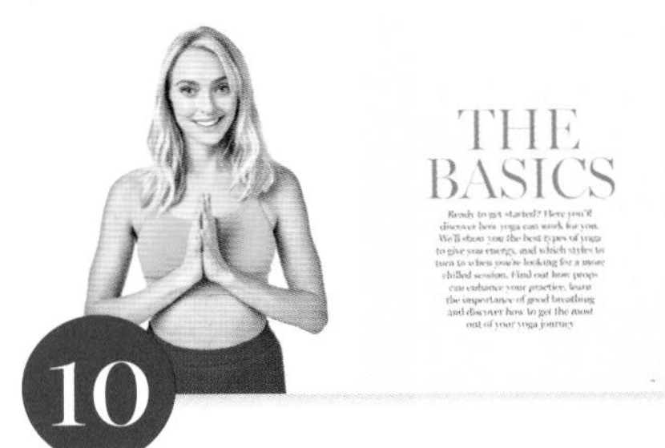

LEARN THE BASICS

We begin with what you need to get started. Learn how to get the most from your practice, discover the best types of yoga to give you energy and which styles leave you calm and rested, and uncover the benefits of breathing well.

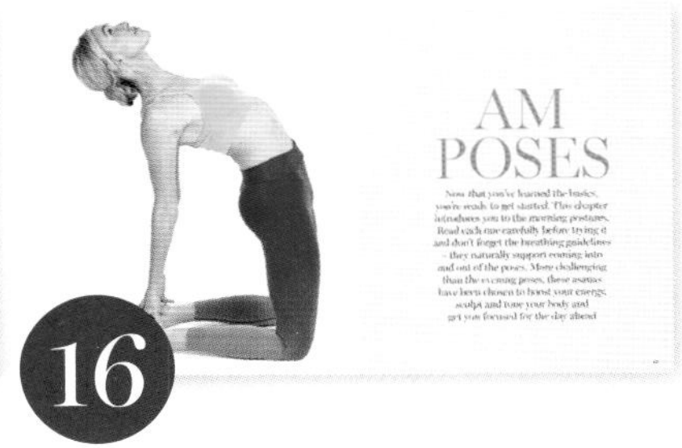

YOUR ENERGY FIX

Learn how to do the energising poses that form the basis of the AM yoga sequences. Each posture comes with in-depth instructions and guidelines for breathing, along with variations and modifications for beginners.

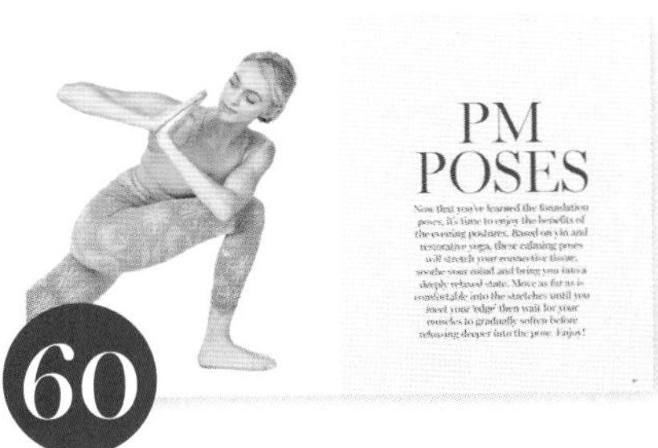

SLOW DOWN

Here we introduce you to a selection of yin and restorative yoga poses that will be used in the PM yoga sessions. You'll learn how to use props, such as bolsters and blocks, and discover ways to deepen your experience of relaxation.

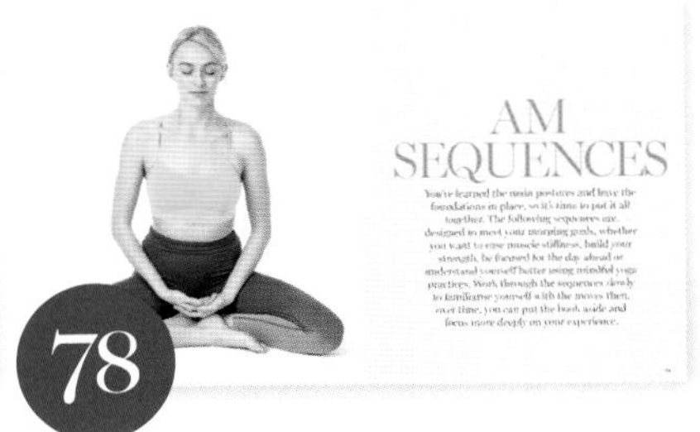

RISE AND SHINE

Now you've learned the foundations, it's time to put everything into practice. In this chapter you'll find AM warm-up poses, sun salutations and morning sequences to give you energy, help you focus and stretch out tight muscles.

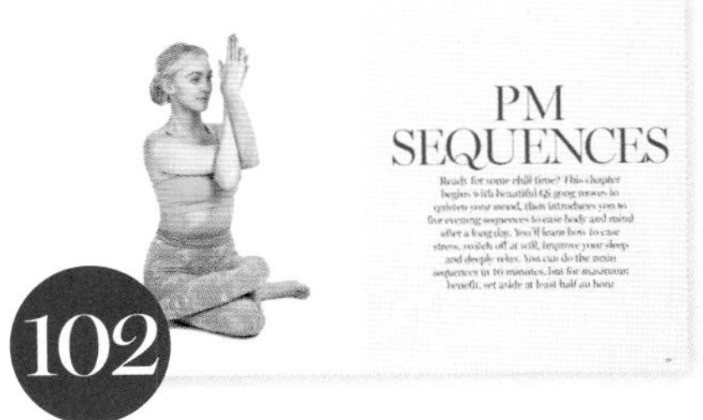

EVENING RITUALS

At the end of a long day, come home to these calming sequences. Soft Qi gong moves, flowing Moon salutes, restorative flows and soothing meditations will refresh you and soothe away the day's stresses.

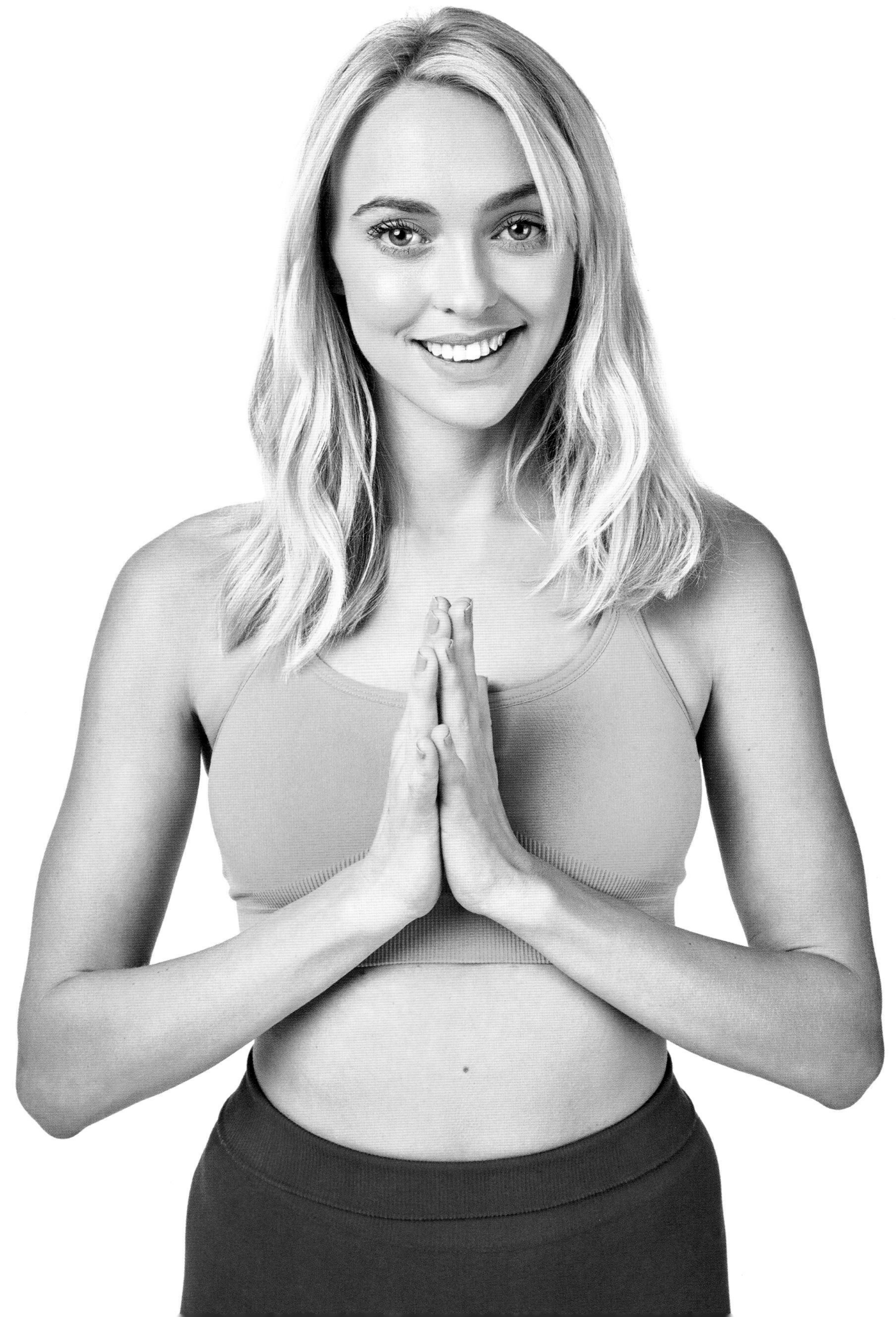

THE BASICS

Ready to get started? Here you'll discover how yoga can work for you. We'll show you the best types of yoga to give you energy, and which styles to turn to when you're looking for a more chilled session. Find out how props can enhance your practice, learn the importance of good breathing and discover how to get the most out of your yoga journey

INTRODUCTION TO YOGA

While energising your body and calming your mind, yoga practice also allows you to achieve a deeper understanding of how you live your life

In our busy, hectic lives, taking time out for self-care is becoming increasingly important. Work deadlines, family commitments, social engagements and a 24/7 social media presence inevitably takes its toll on our bodies and our wellbeing. Fortunately, yoga provides a welcome antidote to 21st century living. Anyone who's ever practised the ancient disciple can tell you of the amazing benefits it brings, from easing stress, to reducing pain, enhancing flexibility, building a strong, toned body and increasing confidence. You can enter a yoga session feeling stressed, with your thoughts racing and your body tense, but in just 10 minutes you'll feel calmer, more relaxed and gently energised. In fact, if you've never done yoga before, the transformation you'll feel will soon have you hooked!

While yoga is having a massive surge in popularity at the moment, its origins date as far back as 5,000BC with the first practical guide written around 2,500 years ago. Called the *The Yoga Sutras*, the Indian author and sage Patañjali described yoga as a practice that could 'calm the fluctuations of the mind'. At that point, yogis used meditation rather than the physical poses we now associate with yoga, but the intention remains the same, to still the chatter of your mind – whether that's by attuning to your breath, meditating or placing your body in specific postures.

AND BREATHE...

Learning to breathe well can make a massive difference to your life. All too often we only use a fraction of our lung capacity, which not only means your muscles receive less oxygen, making yoga postures more difficult to attain, but your brain will be less efficient too. Once you start to explore the different ways to use your breath, including yogic breathing (p122), you can use these skills to ease stress, deeply relax, boost your energy and even aid concentration. This book will introduce you to various yogic breathing techniques to meet your differing day-to-day needs, but in the meantime, these are the main principles to be aware of.

Breathe through your nose: Breathing in and out though your nose allows you to control the speed at which air enters and leaves your body, and how evenly you breathe. This, in turn, creates different effects – increasing the length of your exhale, for example, activates the relaxation response in your nervous system.

Connect with your breath: Your yoga practice won't feel very calming if your thoughts are on tomorrow's 'to do' list. When your mind is wandering, bringing your attention back to your breath will help you stay connected to your body. Or, if you're struggling with a particular posture, a balance pose for example, focusing on your breath will help you stay present and attuned to what your body needs to be doing in the present moment to make the posture more comfortable and sustainable. >

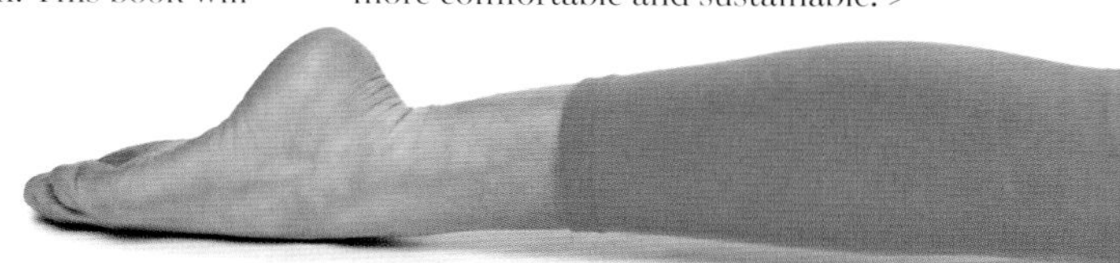

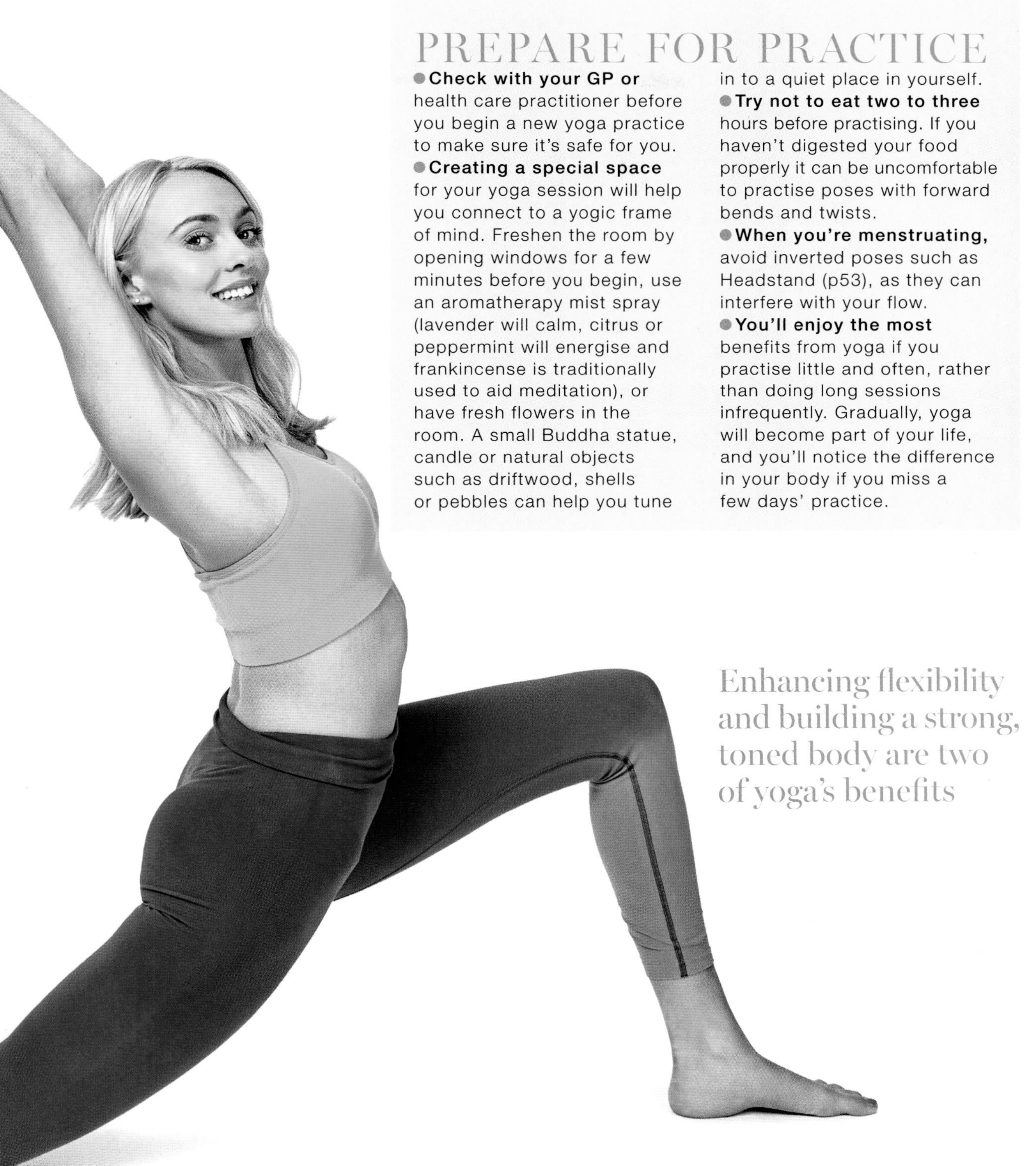

PREPARE FOR PRACTICE

- **Check with your GP or** health care practitioner before you begin a new yoga practice to make sure it's safe for you.
- **Creating a special space** for your yoga session will help you connect to a yogic frame of mind. Freshen the room by opening windows for a few minutes before you begin, use an aromatherapy mist spray (lavender will calm, citrus or peppermint will energise and frankincense is traditionally used to aid meditation), or have fresh flowers in the room. A small Buddha statue, candle or natural objects such as driftwood, shells or pebbles can help you tune in to a quiet place in yourself.
- **Try not to eat two to three** hours before practising. If you haven't digested your food properly it can be uncomfortable to practise poses with forward bends and twists.
- **When you're menstruating,** avoid inverted poses such as Headstand (p53), as they can interfere with your flow.
- **You'll enjoy the most** benefits from yoga if you practise little and often, rather than doing long sessions infrequently. Gradually, yoga will become part of your life, and you'll notice the difference in your body if you miss a few days' practice.

Enhancing flexibility and building a strong, toned body are two of yoga's benefits

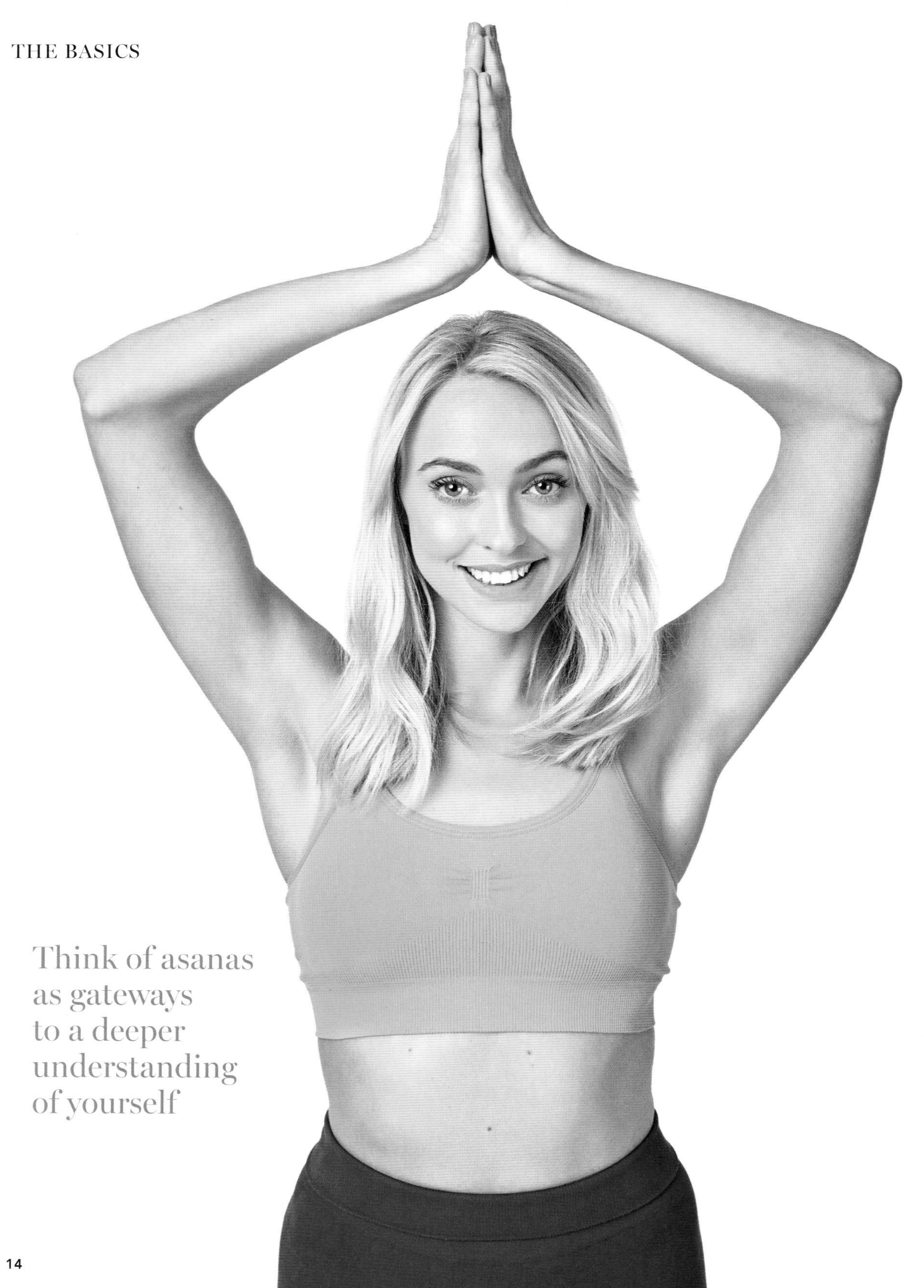

Think of asanas as gateways to a deeper understanding of yourself

Breathe with your movement: The way you breathe as you come into and out of poses, as well as in the sequences, can enhance the benefits you gain. For example, exhaling as you fold your body in Standing forward fold (p52) will help you release into a deeper bend. In general, inhale as you open, lengthen or expand your body or raise an arm or leg, and exhale as you fold forwards or release your limbs. Check out the individual pose instructions for specific guidance.

THE DEEPER BENEFITS OF YOGA

In the poses section (p22-p77) we've described the physical benefits of individual postures, but their benefits go far deeper. Rather than view asanas as static goals to achieve, think of them as gateways to a deeper understanding of yourself. After you've learnt the basics and become more comfortable in the postures, you may be surprised at some of the emotions you feel while practising them. Standing in Warrior II (p56), for example, can connect you with a strength and focus you didn't realise you had. Finding stillness as you balance in Tree (p54) is an experience you can draw on during stressful moments and flood you with feelings of calm.

The main thing to remember initially is to be kind to yourself on the mat – it's a great place to practise being kind to yourself in life. If you force yourself into a posture, or ignore any pain or discomfort you feel while there, you're likely to treat yourself that way off your mat too. Or, if you're more concerned what the person on the mat next to you is thinking of your Downward dog (p30), you may be in danger of living your life to suit other people rather than focusing on following your own path. Let your mat – especially when following the meditations on p100 and p125 – become a sanctuary and a place to learn more about who you are and who you'd like to be.

GET THE MOST FROM YOUR SESSION

- **Always check in with how you're feeling at the beginning of your practice.** Spend a few moments in Mountain pose (p44) or Extended child's pose (p34), breathe into your belly to let your mind begin to quieten and release any tension in the back of your neck and shoulders as you exhale. Notice your thoughts, feelings and bodily sensations, then choose which sequence most meets your needs at the time.
- **After you've gained basic experience, if you're really pushed for time and need a 'quick fix', choose a couple of poses and practise them when you have a few minutes spare.** Opt for forward folds when you want to feel calm and relaxed (try Seated forward fold, p50) and any pose in which you arch your spine backwards for an energising boost (Crescent with arms behind your back, p29). Or follow one of the breathing practices for relaxation (Alternate nostril breathing, p123) or energy (Bellows breath, p99).
- **When you need some extra inspiration, working with a teacher you resonate with can take your practice deeper.** Or, if getting to class is difficult to fit into your schedule, online streaming platforms are a wonderful way to broaden your yoga experience. One of the best, ekhartyoga.com, has many inspiring teachers, and you can choose individual classes (from 10-90 minutes) in many yoga styles or follow programmes to build your strength, sleep better or reduce anxiety.
- **Remember, yoga isn't a competition – with others or yourself.** Rather than trying to recreate what you think a pose is supposed to look like from the outside, tune into your body and feel what the posture is like from the inside. Be sensitive to how your arms are positioned in the space around you, feel if your weight is evenly distributed between your feet, notice how your back feels. This way you'll learn to embody the postures for yourself, rather than copy how someone – with a different physiology to you – does the pose.
- **Setting an intention is a powerful way to focus your practice.** When you check in (see above) or practise meditations spend a moment or two attuning to what you most deeply long for, either for your practice or for your life. Perhaps you want to feel stronger in your body, or maybe you want to stop seeking perfection. Simply allow the feeling to permeate your body and mind and then let it go. Setting an intention in this way slowly creates the space for you to begin to make alternative choices and allows insights to come to you that may help you practise yoga, or live your life, in a different way.

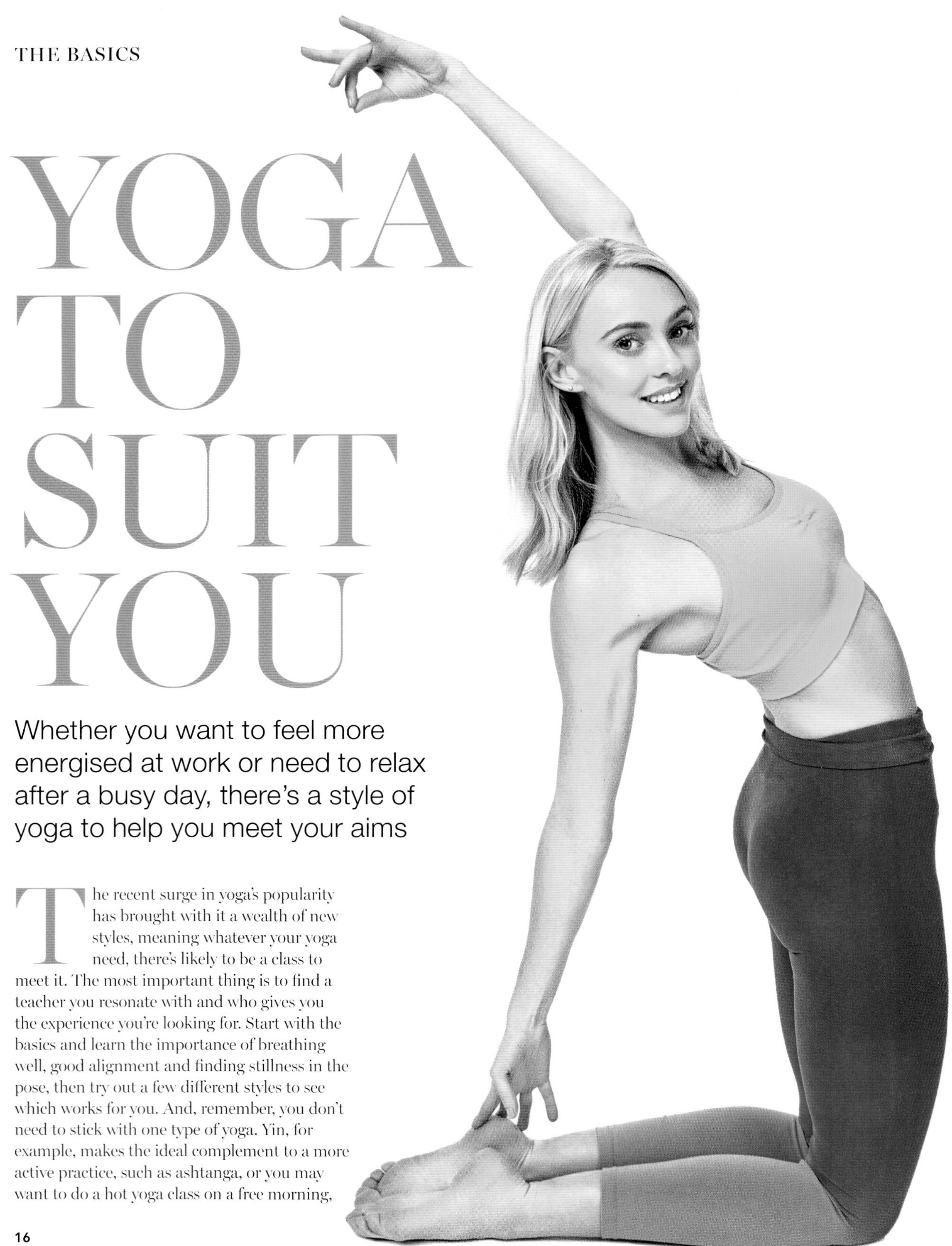

YOGA TO SUIT YOU

Whether you want to feel more energised at work or need to relax after a busy day, there's a style of yoga to help you meet your aims

The recent surge in yoga's popularity has brought with it a wealth of new styles, meaning whatever your yoga need, there's likely to be a class to meet it. The most important thing is to find a teacher you resonate with and who gives you the experience you're looking for. Start with the basics and learn the importance of breathing well, good alignment and finding stillness in the pose, then try out a few different styles to see which works for you. And, remember, you don't need to stick with one type of yoga. Yin, for example, makes the ideal complement to a more active practice, such as ashtanga, or you may want to do a hot yoga class on a free morning, balanced by a calming restorative session at the end of a long and busy week. The following styles have been divided into those that will leave you buzzing and raring to go, and more calming yoga practices to still your mind.

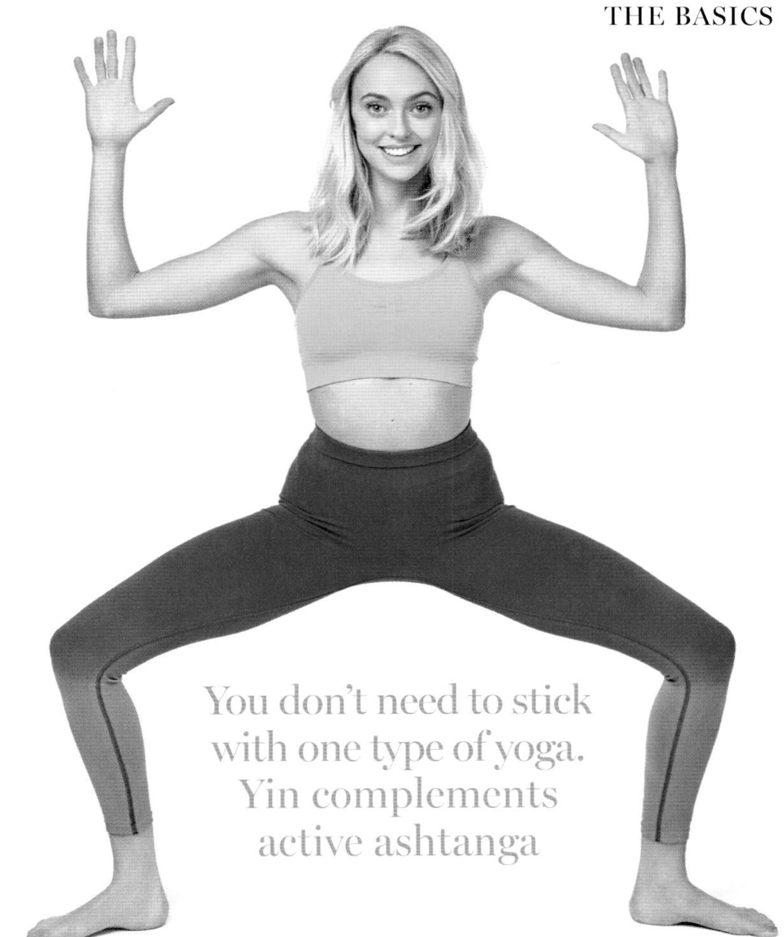

You don't need to stick with one type of yoga. Yin complements active ashtanga

YOGA FOR ENERGY

ASHTANGA

Sometimes referred to as power yoga, ashtanga was brought to the West by Sri K Pattabhi Jois, one of the modern founding fathers of yoga. It's a challenging form and you work through a progressive series of postures before moving on to the next. The Primary Series is said to detoxify and align the body, while the Intermediate Series purifies the nervous system by opening and clearing the energy channels, and so on. Classes often take a 'Mysore' form, with no formal teaching – everyone works at their own pace, while the teacher walks around giving individual guidance as needed. There's no music and little talking – just the sound of energising ujjayi breathing (p98) – enabling you to become absorbed in your practice. Mysore sessions may be up to three hours long, often taking place early in the morning, but you don't have to stay for the whole session, you can drop in at any time and stay as long as is right for you.

GOOD FOR: A light and strong body and a calm mind.

HOT YOGA

Originally developed by Bikram Chaudhury in the 1970s and 80s, this is a challenging form of yoga guaranteed to make you sweat! With studio temperatures ranging from 30-40°C and up to 40 per cent humidity, proponents claim classes have cleansing and detoxifying effects. Sessions are often 90 minutes long, and have both cardio and strength benefits. You'll need to take a towel to class with you, and some students place a thin towel on their mat to prevent slipping when sweat falls onto it. The higher temperatures will make you feel more flexible than usual, but it's important not too push yourself too far or you could end up with an injury. Some studios now use infrared heat which they claim warms the body, rather than the surrounding air, making it a safer option. Remember to take a bottle of water with you – you'll need it!

GOOD FOR: Burning calories, cardio, muscle conditioning.

BOXING YOGA

A newcomer to the yoga scene, this system aims to improve your strength, flexibility and physical health and maximise your performance in other sports. There's little mention of the spiritual aspects of traditional yoga – no chanting, sanskrit pose names or yoga philosphy – the focus is purely on the physical and mental benefits. Classes are around 60-minutes long to up-beat music and include stretching and balances, shadow boxing and work on all the major muscle groups, all building towards an intense flow sequence with an emphasis on alignment, endurance, mobility and strength.

GOOD FOR: Boosting stamina, enhancing confidence, increasing whole-body strength.

JIVAMUKTI

Another relatively new branch of yoga, jivamukti is the vision of artist David Life and dancer Sharon Gannon. Developed in 1984, it consists of vigorous flowing sequences to an invigorating, shifting soundtrack that varies from world music to the spoken word, ragas to Mozart.

The pair chose the name jivamukti (*jiva* means individual soul and *mukti* refers to liberation) to reflect their belief that you can have a beneficial and fulfilling life in the world, yet still attend to the spiritual dimension. More than just physical yoga postures, jivamukti also involves spiritual teachings, meditation and chanting.
GOOD FOR: Discovering how to take the benefits of yoga off your mat and into your life .

YOGA FOR RELAXATION

YIN

Yin yoga is a quiet, still practice created by Qi gong expert, Paulie Zink, and later developed by Paul Grillie and Sarah Powers. The postures are designed to work your connective tissue, fascia, ligaments, joints and bones, rather than your muscles, and poses are static – mostly sitting or lying down – and held for long periods of time (three to five minutes). The theory behind yin yoga is based on Eastern attitudes to health, and its proponents believe the poses help bring about health by stimulating the meridians and removing energy blocks in the body.
GOOD FOR: Calming your mind, easing anxiety, increasing mindfulness.

SIVANANDA

More than just a physical system, sivananda yoga has a strong spiritual element, and includes breathing, relaxation, diet, positive thinking and meditation. A typical class includes pranayama (breathing exercises), sun salutes, 12 postures and deep relaxation. The poses are practised in the same order each time to systematically work the body in a way that enhances the flow of prana, or life force energy, and with the aim of stilling the mind. Physical benefits include increasing the flexibility of your spine, strengthening your bones and stimulating your circulatory and immune systems.
GOOD FOR: Reducing stress, increasing overall health and reducing the risk of illness.

RESTORATIVE

When you're feeling exhausted, either physically or emotionally, restorative yoga is a wonderful way to soothe a stressed nervous system. Like yin yoga, the poses are mostly seated or lying down, but held for even longer periods - up to 20 minutes - to allow your body to enter a state of deep relaxation. There are a lot of props in restorative yoga, such as bolsters, blankets, blocks, straps, each used to provide maximum support to your body. The theory is that by taking the strain out of the pose, your muscles can fully release. It's important that you're completely comfortable in the poses, so it's worth setting up your props carefully before you get into the posture, and make any adjustments you need before you settle into them.
GOOD FOR: Relieving the physical symptoms of stress, easing insomnia, providing support after emotional turmoil.

ANUSARA

Anusara means 'flowing with grace', and the yoga style has a strong spiritual element. The founder, John Friend, broke away from the movement in 2012, but the remaining teachers continued, forming the Anusara School of Hatha Yoga. Classes begin with an invocation, and are based around a heart-opening theme, with each posture linked to a precise set of alignment principles that emphasise core stability and spinal mobility, sequenced in a fluid way. There are around 250 different asanas, and you'll be encouraged to practise different variations as an expression of your unique spirit. Classes include breathing exercises, chanting, music, mudras (hand gestures) and a focus on the chakras, or energy centres in your body.
GOOD FOR: Lifting your mood, freeing your spine and living your yoga away from the mat.

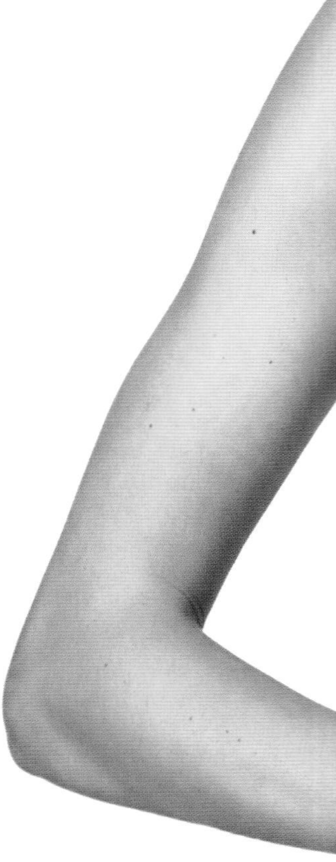

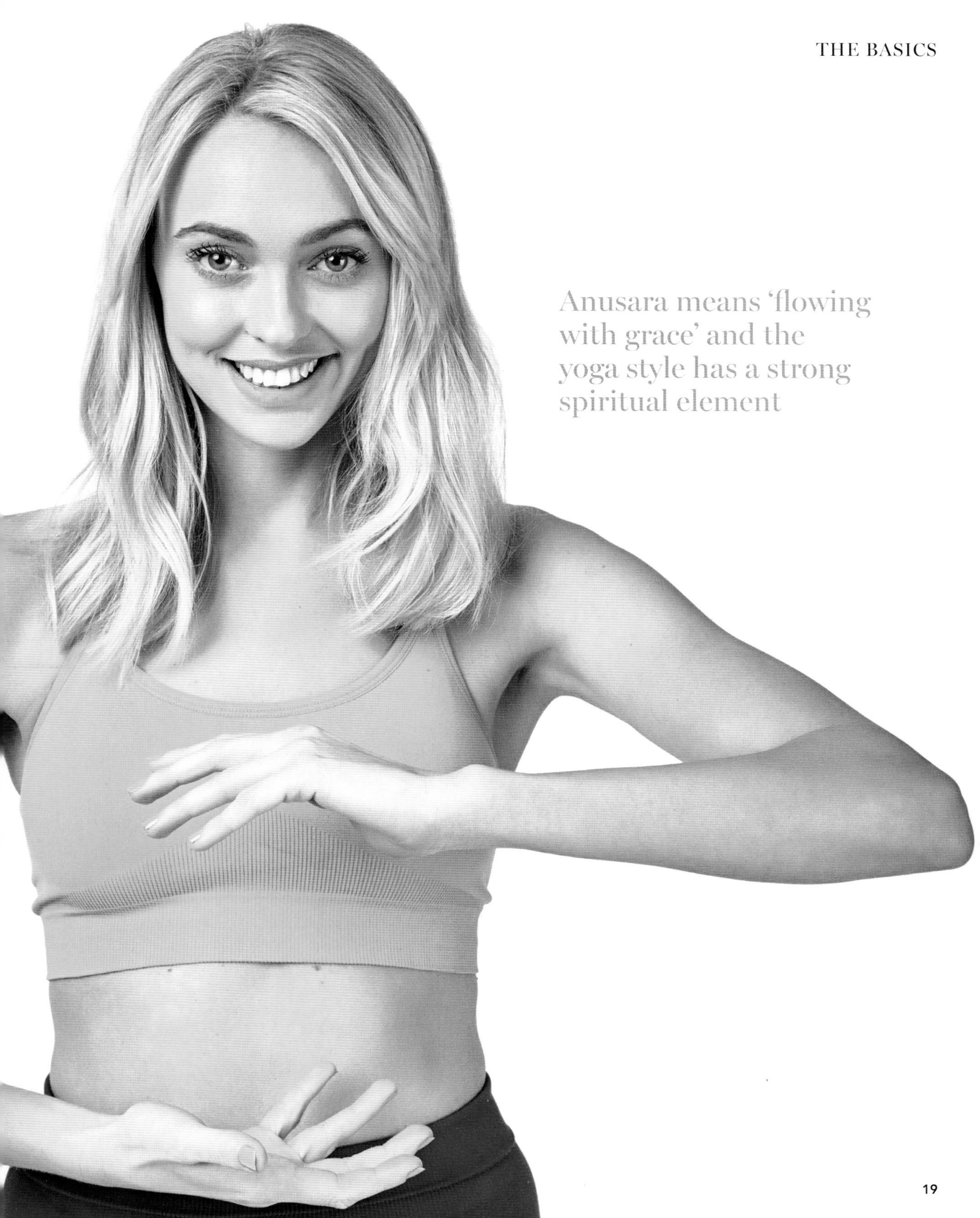

Anusara means 'flowing with grace' and the yoga style has a strong spiritual element

WHAT YOU NEED

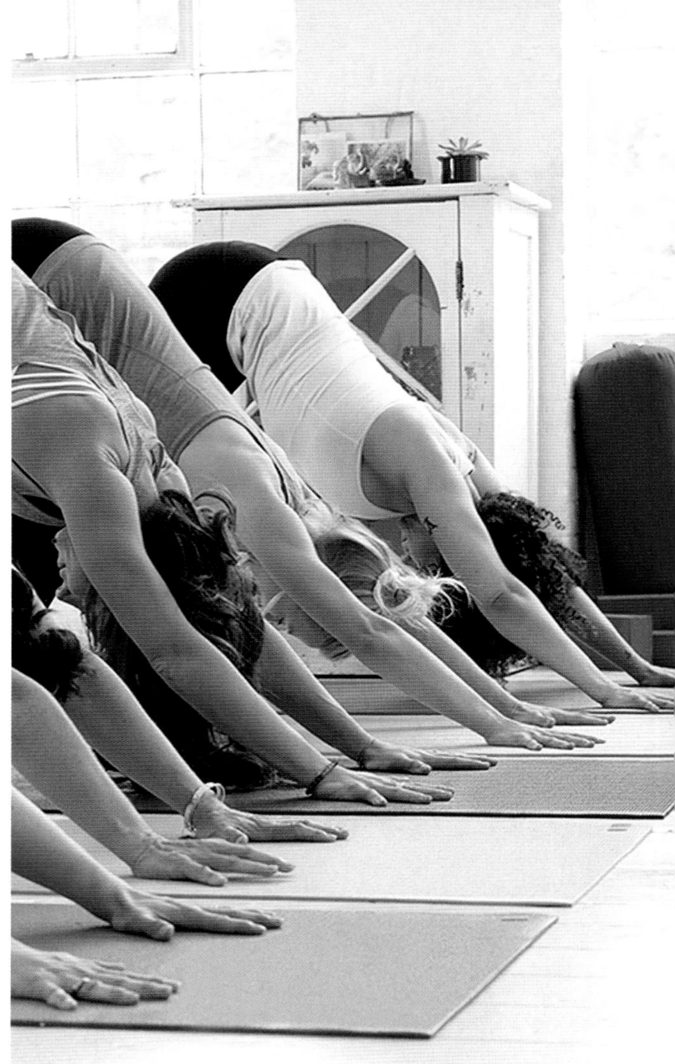

One of the beauties of yoga is that you don't need to buy a lot of equipment – a non-slip mat and comfortable, stretchy clothing will be perfectly fine. But there are a few props that will enable you to get even more out of your practice. Designed to help you experience the benefits of yoga without having to strain or push your self too quickly, too soon, a few well-chosen props will enhance your enjoyment of yoga no end.

1. MAT

Often called a sticky mat, a yoga mat stops your hands and feet from slipping when you're in poses such as Downward dog (p30). They vary in size, thickness and price – you can pay as little as £10 or as much as £100 plus – but as long as they are comfortable to use, you don't need to spend a lot of money on one.
TRY THIS: Yogamatters Sticky Yoga Mat, £17; yogamatters.com

2. BRICKS

A brick is used as an extension of your arms in standing poses, such as Half moon (p38), letting you reach the floor with correct alignment even if you don't have full flexibility or perfect balance. You can also place a brick between your knees in poses such as Chair (p27) or Bridge (p25), to activate your outer thighs. They are made with cork, wood or high-density foam.
TRY THIS: Yogamatters Yoga Brick, £6.50.

3. BOLSTER

Bolsters support your body in restorative poses, allowing you to relax deeply. Cylindrical bolsters are ideal for using under your knees, but if you only want one, you may find a rectangular version more useful. With a larger, flatter surface it's ideal for postures such as Reclining butterfly (p62), where you lie on your back, as well as for raising your hips for long periods of sitting in meditation. Chose one with a machine washable outer cover.
TRY THIS: Yogamatters Rectangular Bolster, £38.

4. BLOCKS

Blocks are thinner and larger than bricks and are a useful way to support, stabilise and align your body. One of their

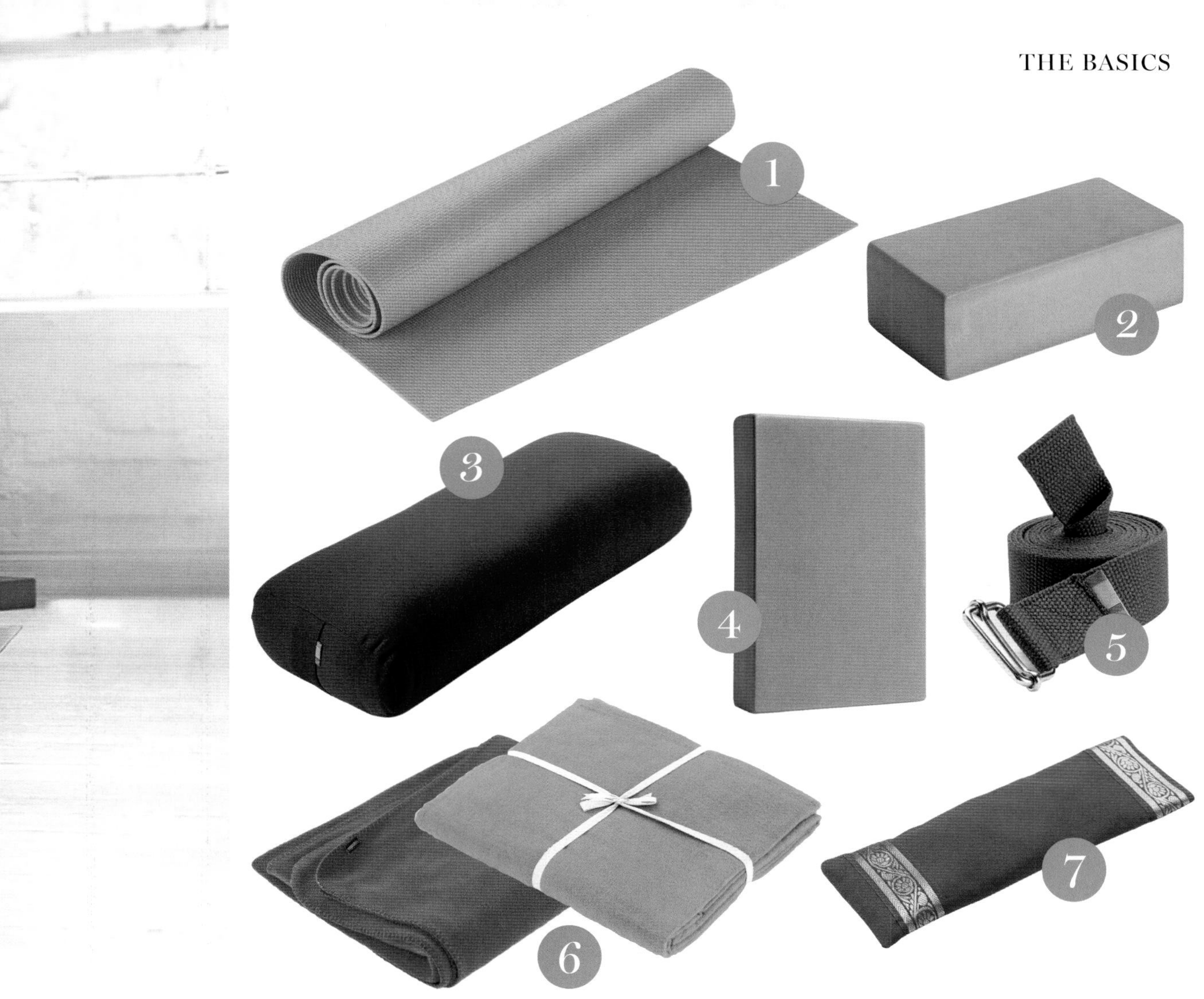

most common uses is for sitting on to raise your hips for a straighter spine in seated postures such as Easy pose (p33).
TRY THIS: Yomagatters Yoga Block, £5.50.

5. STRAP

Popular in lyengar yoga classes, straps can help enhance your alignment before you develop good flexibility. Try wrapping a strap around the balls of your feet and holding one end in each hand for Seated forward fold (p50).
TRY THIS: Yogamatters Wide Yoga Belt, £7.20.

6. BLANKETS

When you've finished an active class, your body temperature rapidly drops when you become still, so a soft blanket is ideal to keep you warm for the relaxation or meditation section. In restorative yoga poses such as those you'll find in the PM section of the book, a firm blanket is used to rest and support your head, neck and limbs to aid the deepest relaxation. You can also lie on folded firm blankets to raise your chest or support your knees when a bolster is too high.

TRY THIS: Yogamatters Coloured Cotton Blanket (firm), £24, and Fleece Yoga Blanket (soft), £25.

7. EYE PILLOW

Even with your eyes closed, light can be a distraction during your relaxation. The gentle pressure of a pillow on your eyes releases tension in your face, and if you choose one with lavender inside, you'll feel even more soothed.
TRY THIS: Yogamalai Eye Pillow With Lavender, £8; yogamatters.com

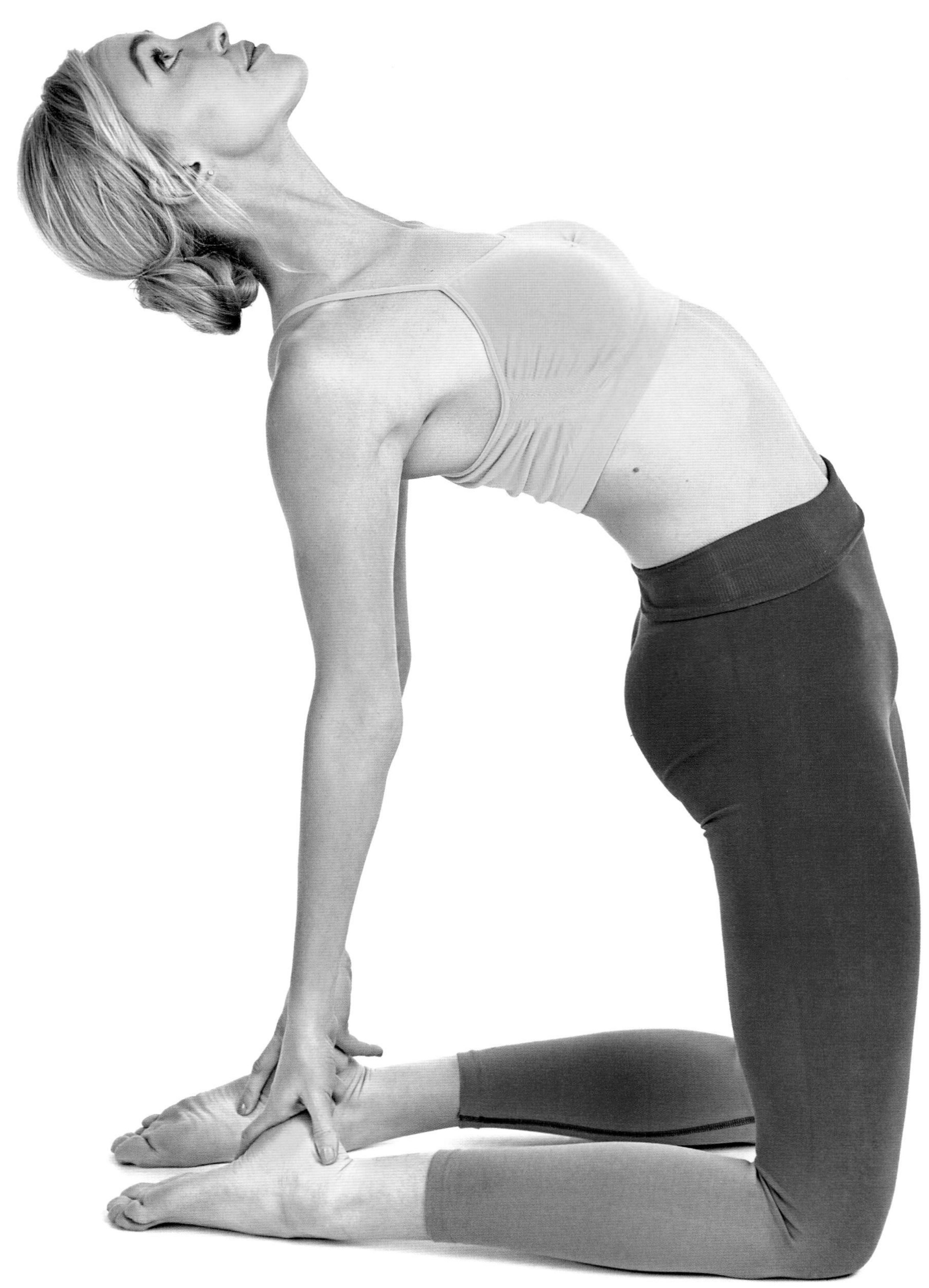

AM POSES

Now that you've learned the basics, you're ready to get started. This chapter introduces you to the morning postures. Read each one carefully before trying it and don't forget the breathing guidelines – they naturally support coming into and out of the poses. More challenging than the evening poses, these asanas have been chosen to boost your energy, sculpt and tone your body and get you focused for the day ahead

BOAT POSE

NAVASANA

- Sit on your mat, bend your knees, raise your feet off the floor and grasp the back of your thighs with your hands.
- Draw your navel to your spine and lean back to balance on your sitting bones. Take a few breaths here, then raise your lower legs until your shins are parallel to the floor.
- If you are comfortable here, extend your arms and hold them parallel to the floor. Take another few breaths, and, if you feel balanced, straighten your legs to take your body into a 'V' shape with your arms lifted higher and your palms facing the ceiling.
- Draw your shoulder blades down your spine and keep your abdominals engaged, with your feet relaxed. Take up to five breaths before releasing on an exhale.

GOOD FOR

- Aids focus
- Eases stress
- Tones your abdominals
- Strengthens your back muscles

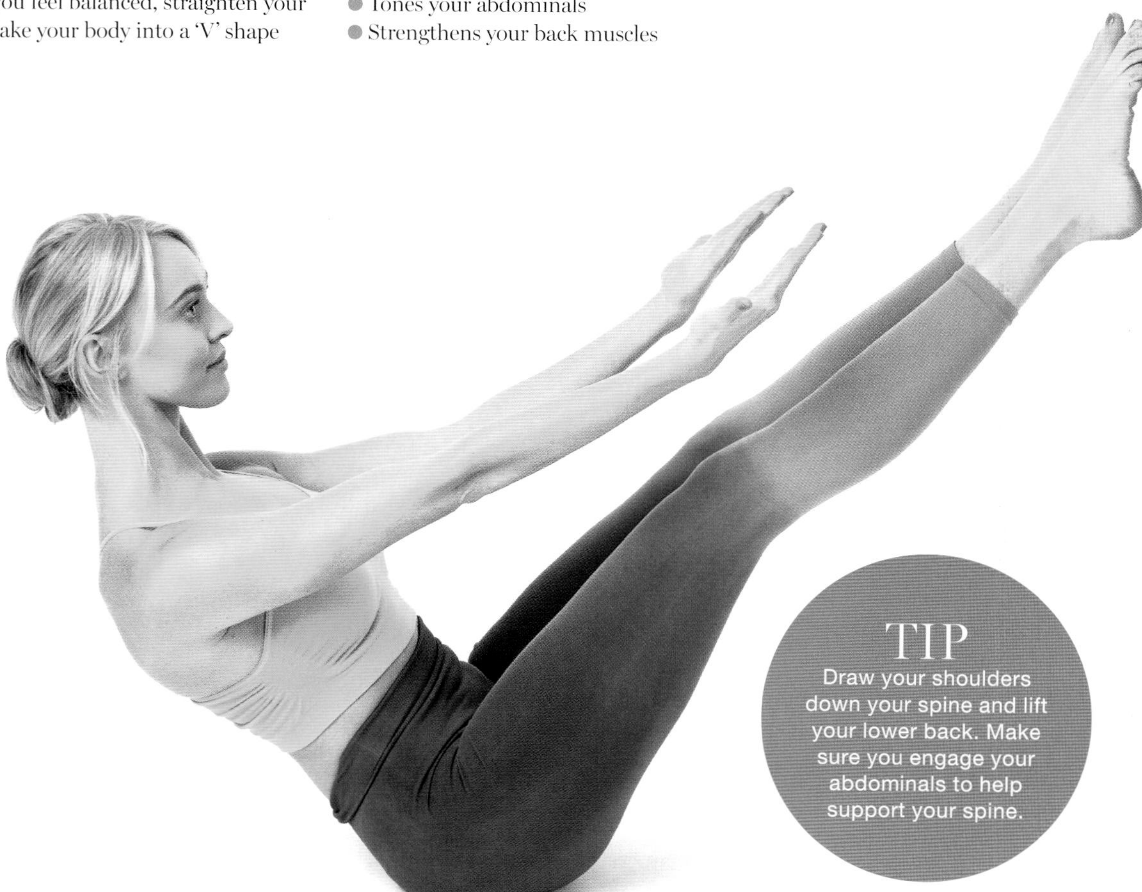

TIP

Draw your shoulders down your spine and lift your lower back. Make sure you engage your abdominals to help support your spine.

BRIDGE POSE
SETU BANDHA SARVANGASANA

● Lie on your back, bend your knees and place your feet hip-distance apart and parallel, directly beneath your knees. Rest your arms at your sides, palms facing down.

● Inhale, ground through your feet and, on an exhale, tilt your tailbone up to gently peel your spine away from the floor, vertebra by vertebra.

● Keep your thighs parallel, knees hip-distance apart, and continue rooting through your feet to lift your chest. Roll your shoulders up, back and down, then lengthen the back of your neck.

● Bring your hands together beneath you, interlink your fingers and snuggle your shoulders together (A). Focus on grounding through your feet to lift through your heart.

● Take five deep breaths into your abdomen then, on an exhale, slowly uncurl your spine to rest on the floor.

GOOD FOR

● Boosts your nervous system
● Calms your brain
● Rests your heart
● Helps reduce insomnia

VARIATION (B)

● Once in the pose, draw your right knee to your chest, then lengthen your leg, reaching your toes towards the ceiling. Take three to five deep breaths, lower, then repeat on the other side.

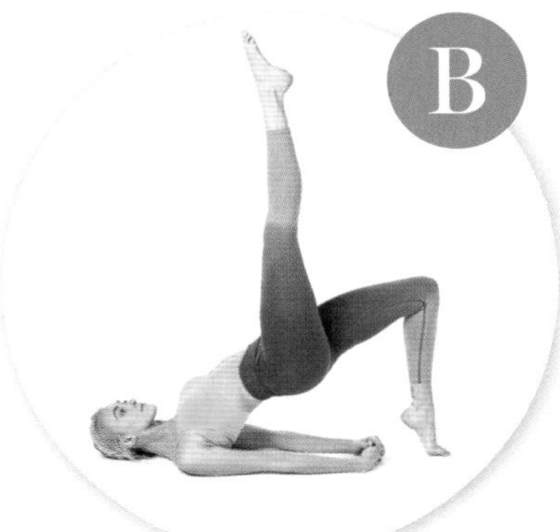

TIP

If your knees tend to splay outwards, practise with a foam block between your thighs to help you engage your inner thigh muscles.

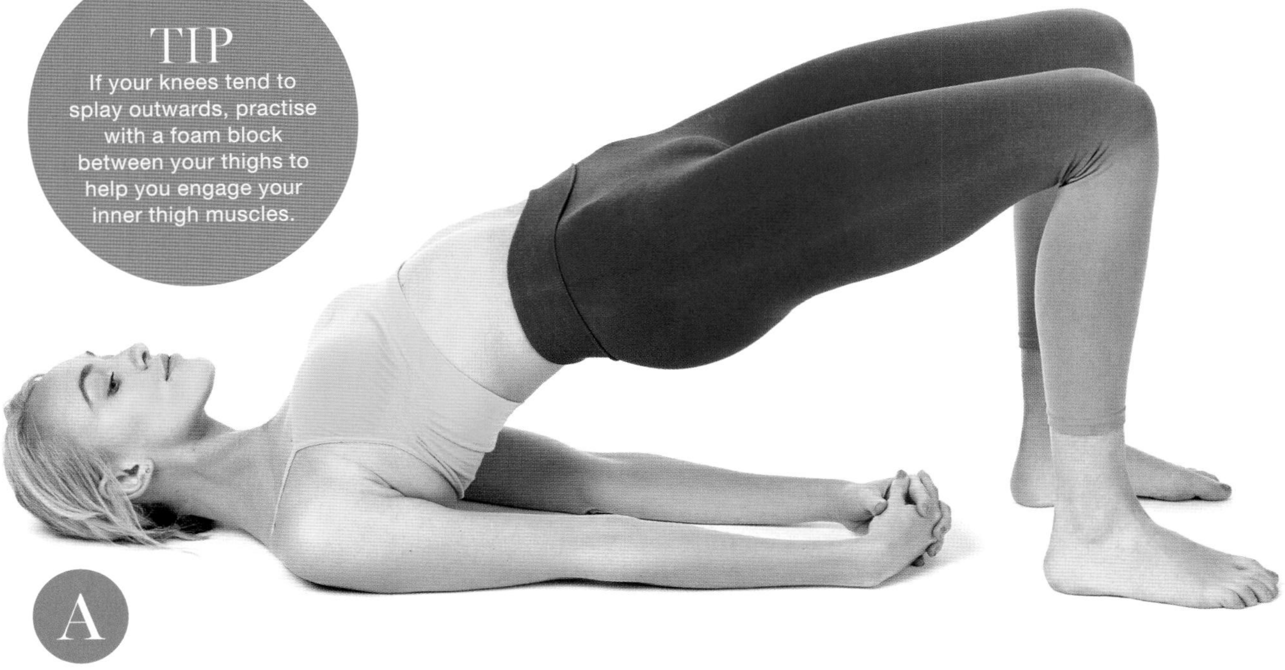

A

CAMEL
USTRASANA

- Kneel on a mat with your thighs hip-width apart, and the front of your toes resting on the mat.
- Inhale, lengthen your spine and circle your left arm over head and rest it on your left ankle, fingers pointing to the soles of your feet. Exhale.
- On your next inhale, repeat the same move with your right hand, eyes looking ahead so you don't strain your neck. Exhale.
- As you inhale, lift your sternum gently upwards, opening your chest and shoulders. Release your tailbone towards the floor to feel the stretch in your quads and core.
- Maintain the length in your neck, and tuck your chin in slightly.
- Take five to 10 deep breaths, then release on an exhale and rest in Child's pose (p34).

GOOD FOR
- Boosts energy
- Deep chest and heart opener
- Strengthens your thighs
- Opens your hip flexors

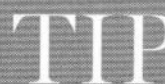

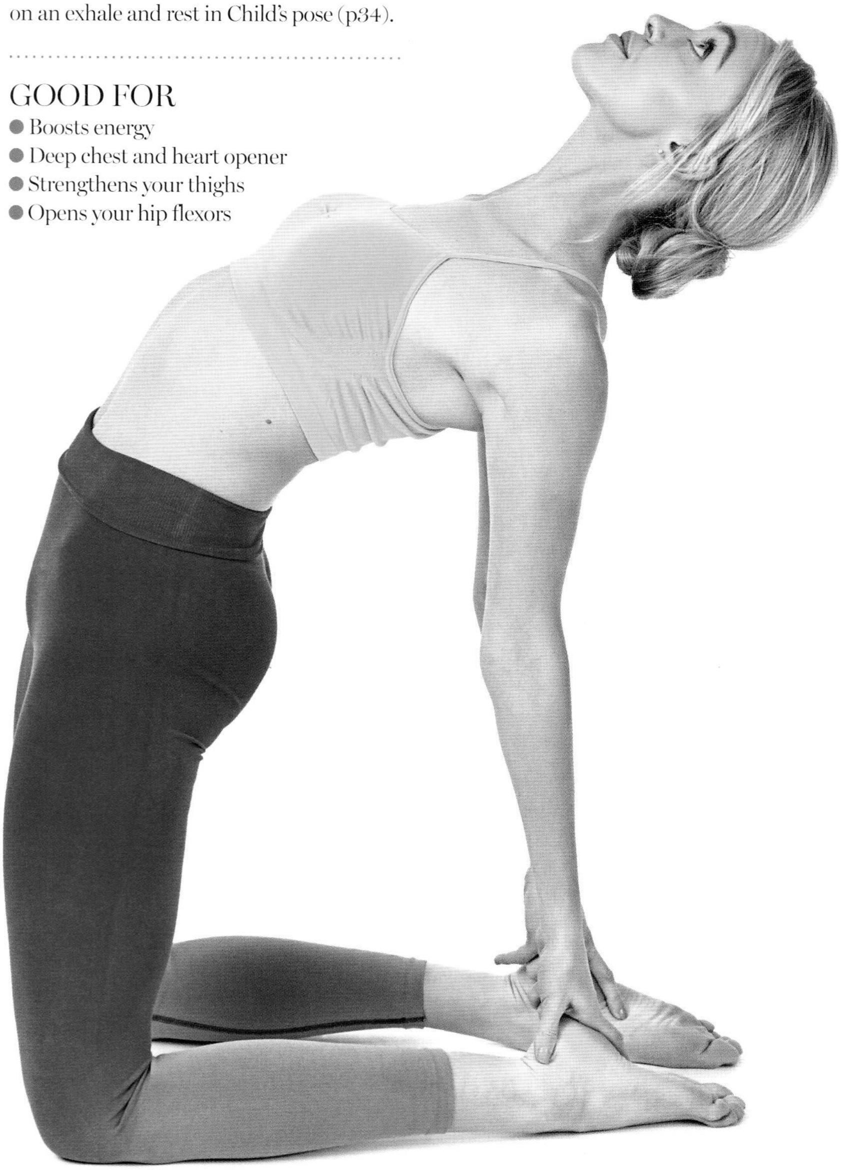

TIP
If this pose is challenging for you, practise with your toes turned under and your hands on blocks either side of your ankles.

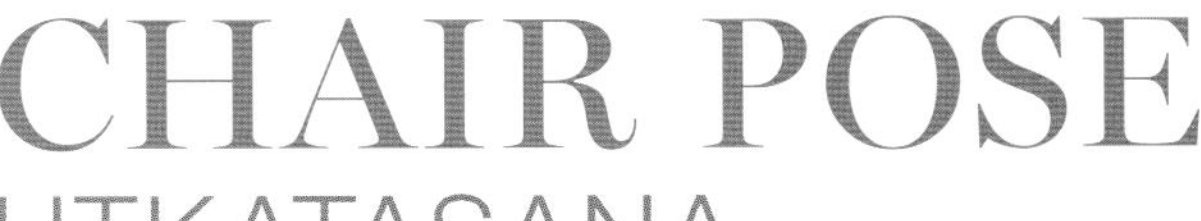

CHAIR POSE
UTKATASANA

● Stand with your feet hip-width apart and fold forwards from your hips, letting your arms hang by your sides.
● Bend your knees deeply, making sure your knees don't extend beyond your toes, then take your arms backwards and look forwards. On an inhale, ground through the base of your big and little toes, and sweep your arms up and forwards, palms facing, until your upper arms are level with your ears.
● Engage your core by drawing your belly button to your spine and allow your shoulder blades to release down your back. Lengthen your spine and extend through to your fingertips, at the same time as drawing your arms into your shoulder sockets. Keep your neck in line with your spine (A).
● Take five breaths, rooting and lengthening through to your fingertips on an inhale; sinking a little deeper on each exhale.

VARIATION
CHAIR TWIST (B)

● In chair pose, imagine you are drawing your thighbones into your hip sockets – this will anchor your pelvis and enable you to twist more deeply. Bring your hands into prayer position at your chest, then inhale to lengthen your spine. As you exhale, twist to the right and balance your outer left elbow against your outer right thigh. Press your palms together and use the leverage of your left arm against your right thigh to gently deepen the twist, making sure your elbow doesn't push your knees out of alignment. Repeat on the other side.

GOOD FOR
● Stretches your shoulders and chest
● Strengthens your legs and spine
● Stimulates your heart
● Stabilising

TIP
Place a block or thick book between your thighs to strengthen your legs even more.

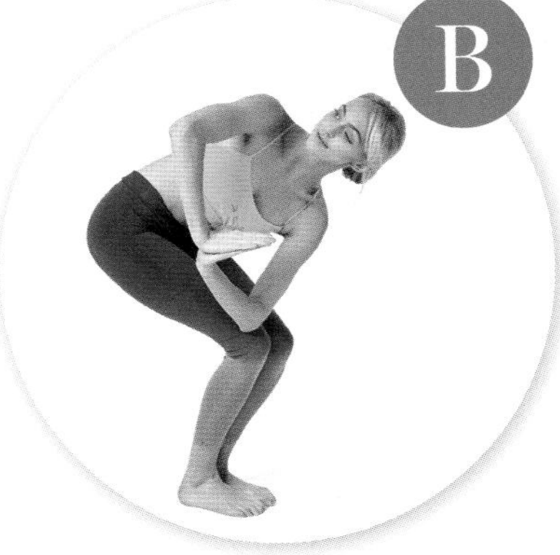

COBRA
BHUJANGASANA

TIP
If this pose feels challenging, take your hands wider apart and turn your wrists outwards. If you are comfortable, straighten your arms to raise your chest higher.

- Lie on your stomach with your forehead resting on the floor. Take a couple of deep breaths, then spread your feet hip-distance apart, ankles straight and toes spread. Straighten your legs, aligning your knees with your middle toes, and engage your inner leg muscles, lifting your inner thighs up and out. Root through your pubic bone.
- Place your hands beneath your shoulders, palms facing down, fingers spread and wrist crease parallel with the front edge of your mat. Root through the base of your thumbs and index fingers.
- Draw your elbows together and rotate your shoulders up, back and down to create space at the base of your neck, then release your shoulder blades down your back and in towards your spine.
- Engage your abdomen and root through your pelvic bone to extend your sacrum to your tailbone.
- Inhale, and raise your head and shoulders as far as is comfortable by drawing the back of your neck upwards, so your eyes remain looking down (A). Exhale.
- On an inhale, ground through your hands, as if you were pulling the floor towards you, and feel your chest open as you curl your spine further forwards and up.
- Lengthen your spine evenly without compressing the back of your neck or your lumbar spine, and see if you can feel a sense of lightness as you lift your back body.
- Breathe normally in the pose for three to five breaths. Slowly and with control, exhale as you lower your body to the floor one vertebra at a time, and rest your head on one side.

GOOD FOR
- Strengthens your spine, tones your spinal nerves
- Eases tension in your back, shoulders and neck
- Helps relieve stress and fatigue
- Opens your heart and lungs

VARIATION
SPONTANEOUS FLOWING COBRA (B) & (C)
- For a free-form variation, rise up and down a few times, allowing your upper spine and shoulders to move in a fluid spontaneous way. For example, look to the right, tilting your shoulders and upper body to the right (B), then to the left (C), releasing any stiffness and tension as you do so. Come up into full Cobra, then lower to the floor on an exhale and rest for a couple of breaths.

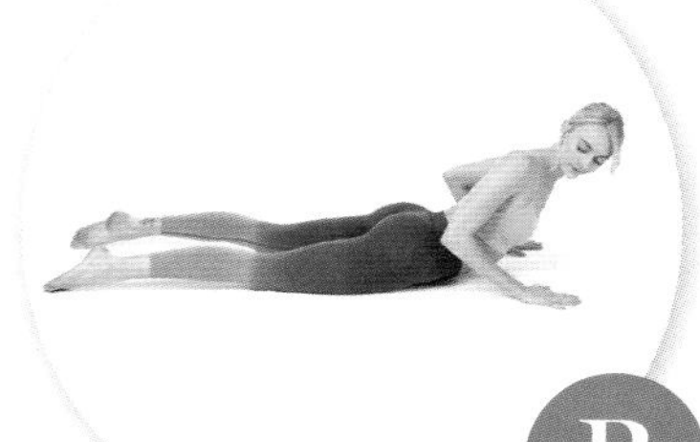
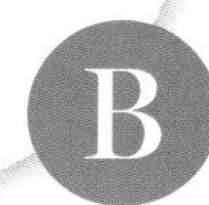

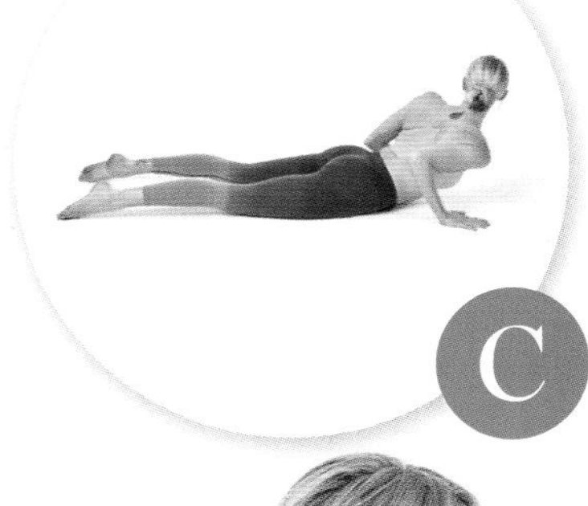

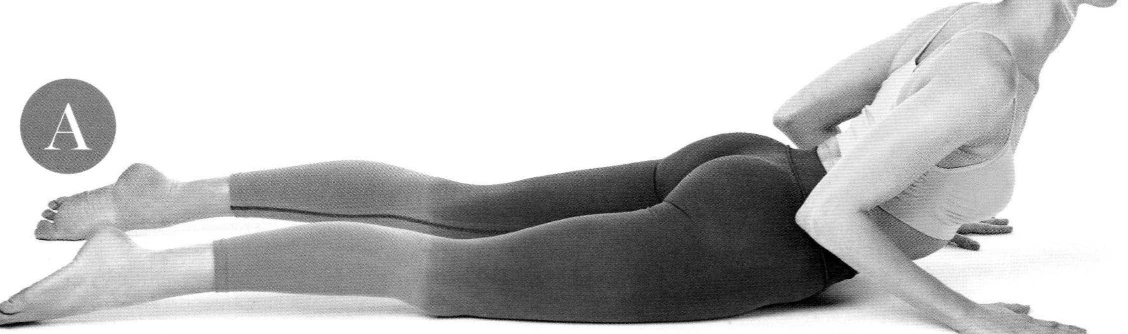

CRESCENT POSE
ANJANEYASANA

- From standing, fold forwards and place your hands either side of your feet. Slide your left leg back and lower onto your knee and the top of your foot. Adjust your right foot, if needed, so your knee is over your ankle. Spread your right toes and lift your inner arch.
- Inhale and raise your torso to vertical, tucking under your tailbone, squaring your hips and drawing your navel towards your spine. As you exhale, sink into your hips.
- Interlace your fingers and thumbs, index fingers pointing forwards, and inhale as you bring your arms over your head (A).
- Take five to 10 deep breaths into your belly, then lower your hands and place either side of your front foot. Step forwards with your back foot and slowly uncurl your spine to return to standing. Repeat on the other side.

VARIATION (B)

- Take your hands behind your back, interlace your fingers and thumbs, and extend your arms backwards and upwards. On each inhale, root down as you lift your chest and arch a little further into the backbend. Exhale as you reach your arms up and back, releasing your shoulder blades down your back. Take five to 10 deep breaths into your belly.

GOOD FOR

- Balance
- Gently energises
- Strengthens your legs
- Opens your hip flexors

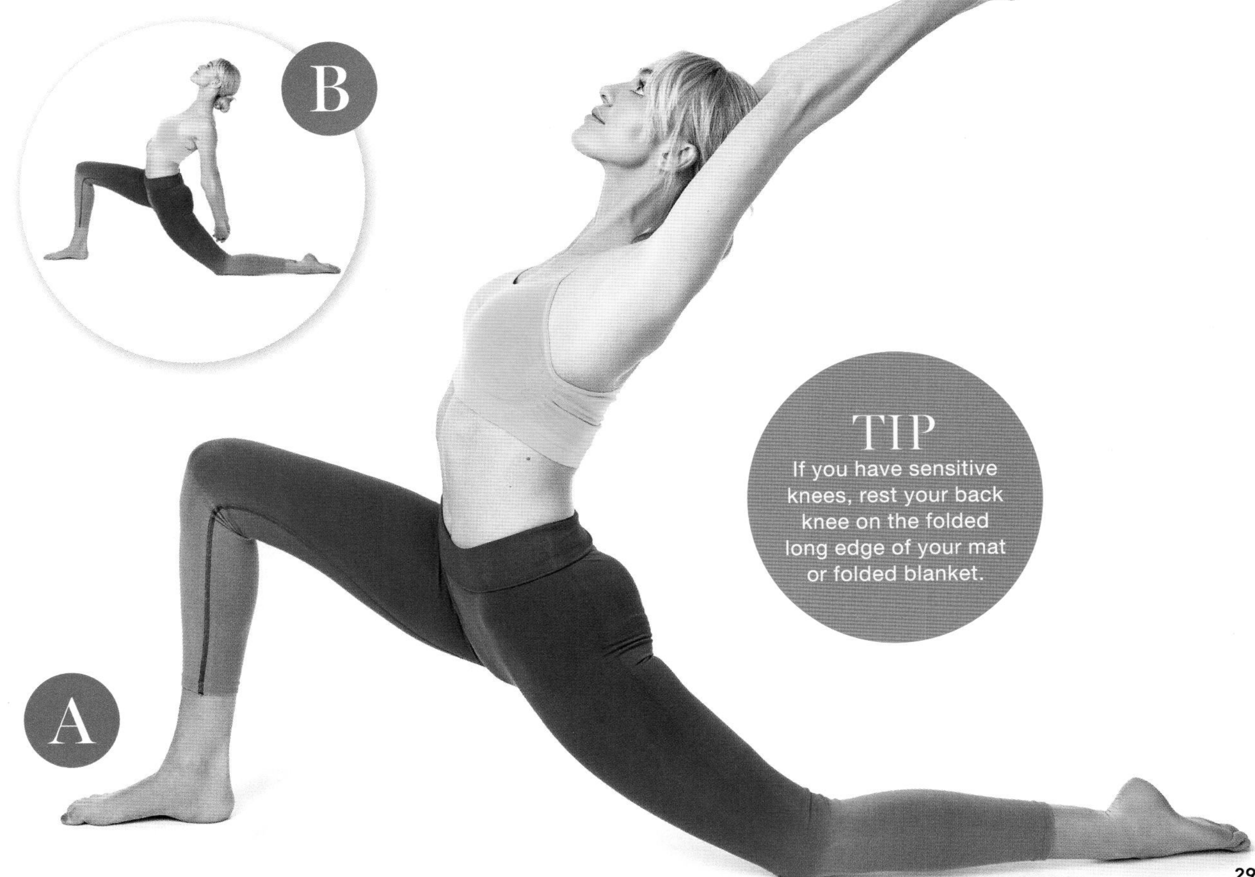

TIP

If you have sensitive knees, rest your back knee on the folded long edge of your mat or folded blanket.

DOWNWARD DOG
ADHO MUKHA SVANASANA

● Start on all fours, knees beneath your hips, and place your hands a palm's length in front of your shoulders, shoulder-width apart and fingers spread.
● Root through the base of your thumbs and index fingers, tuck under your toes and raise your knees off the mat, taking your tailbone back and up to lengthen your spine.
● Keeping your knees bent, root through your hands to extend your spine. Rotate your upper arms externally and draw your shoulder blades down your spine. Lower your front ribs towards your thighs and release your neck.
● Gently draw one heel and then the other towards the mat, stretching out your hamstrings in a walking motion.
● Spread your toes and lower both heels towards the mat. Check that your weight is evenly distributed through each foot and your inner arches are lifted (A).
● Take five deep breaths, then exhale and lower into Child's pose (p34).

GOOD FOR
● Insomnia
● Fatigue
● Calms your nervous system
● Eases palpitations

VARIATION
DOLPHIN POSE (B)
● From kneeling, rest your forearms on the floor, elbows shoulder-width apart. Exhale, tuck under your toes and, pressing your forearms into the floor, raise your knees and straighten your legs. Slowly walk your feet towards your elbows, lifting your tailbone towards the ceiling. Draw your navel to your spine, your shoulders away from your ears and your heels towards the floor. Take five deep breaths, then gently lower.

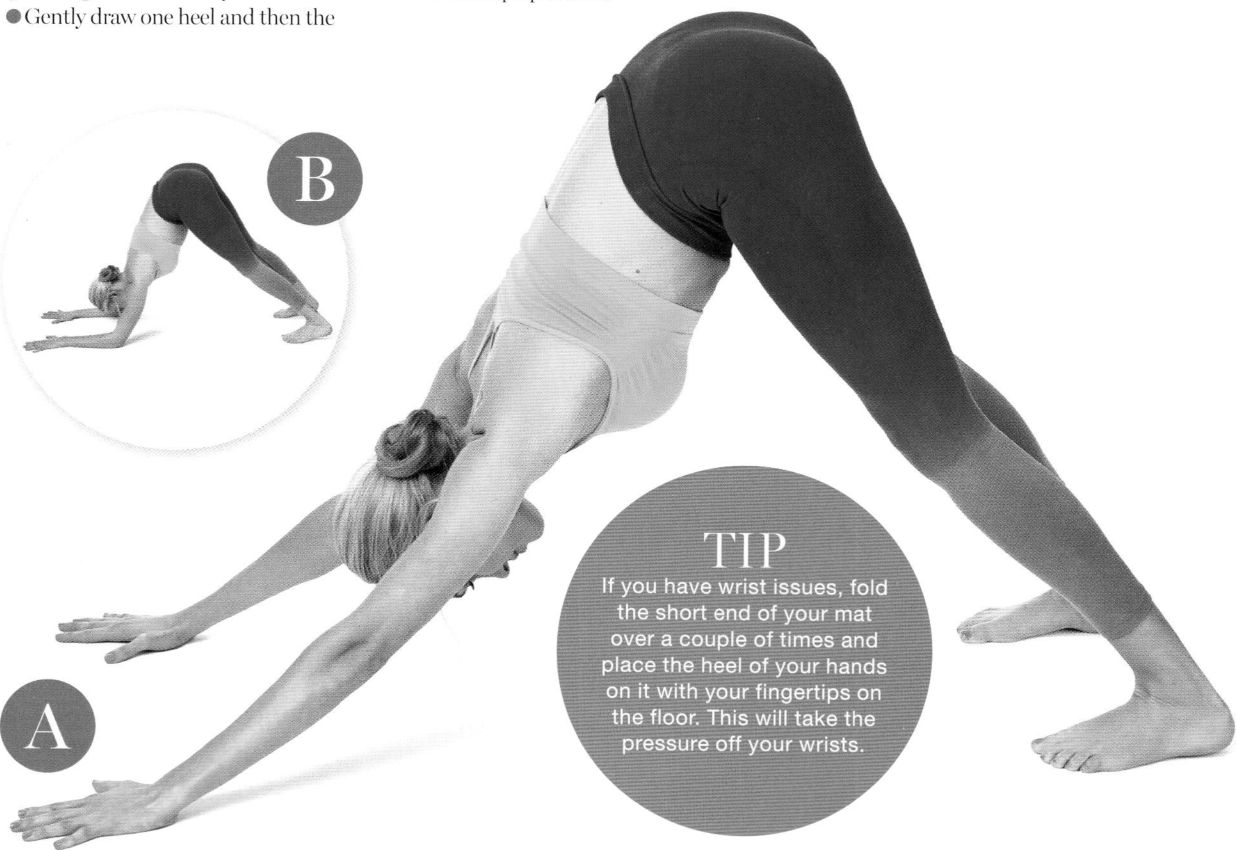

TIP
If you have wrist issues, fold the short end of your mat over a couple of times and place the heel of your hands on it with your fingertips on the floor. This will take the pressure off your wrists.

DOWNWARD DOG SPLITS
EKA PADA ADHO MUKHA SVANASANA

● From Downward dog (p30) step your feet together then, inhale as you sweep your right leg back and up, lifting from your hip. Draw your right hip forwards and your left hip backwards to keep your pelvis square, and internally rotate your raised leg, so your knee and the top of your foot point down towards the mat.

● Root through the base of your thumbs and index fingers, and externally rotate your upper arms. Draw your shoulder blades away from each other and down your spine to create space around your neck.

● Continue lengthening your spine evenly through both sides of your waist and extend your right leg further, to create a straight line from your crown right through to your raised foot (A).

● After five deep breaths, exhale as you lower your leg. Pause for a moment, then repeat on the other side.

VARIATION
DYNAMIC DOWNWARD DOG SPLITS (B)

● For an energising boost, on an exhale, lower your head and draw your raised knee to your chest. Inhale to extend your leg back and up and raise your head again. This is one round. Move mindfully for five rounds, then swap legs.

GOOD FOR

● As for Downward dog, plus:

● Improves your balance

● Opens your ribs to aid breathing

● Releases tension in your hips

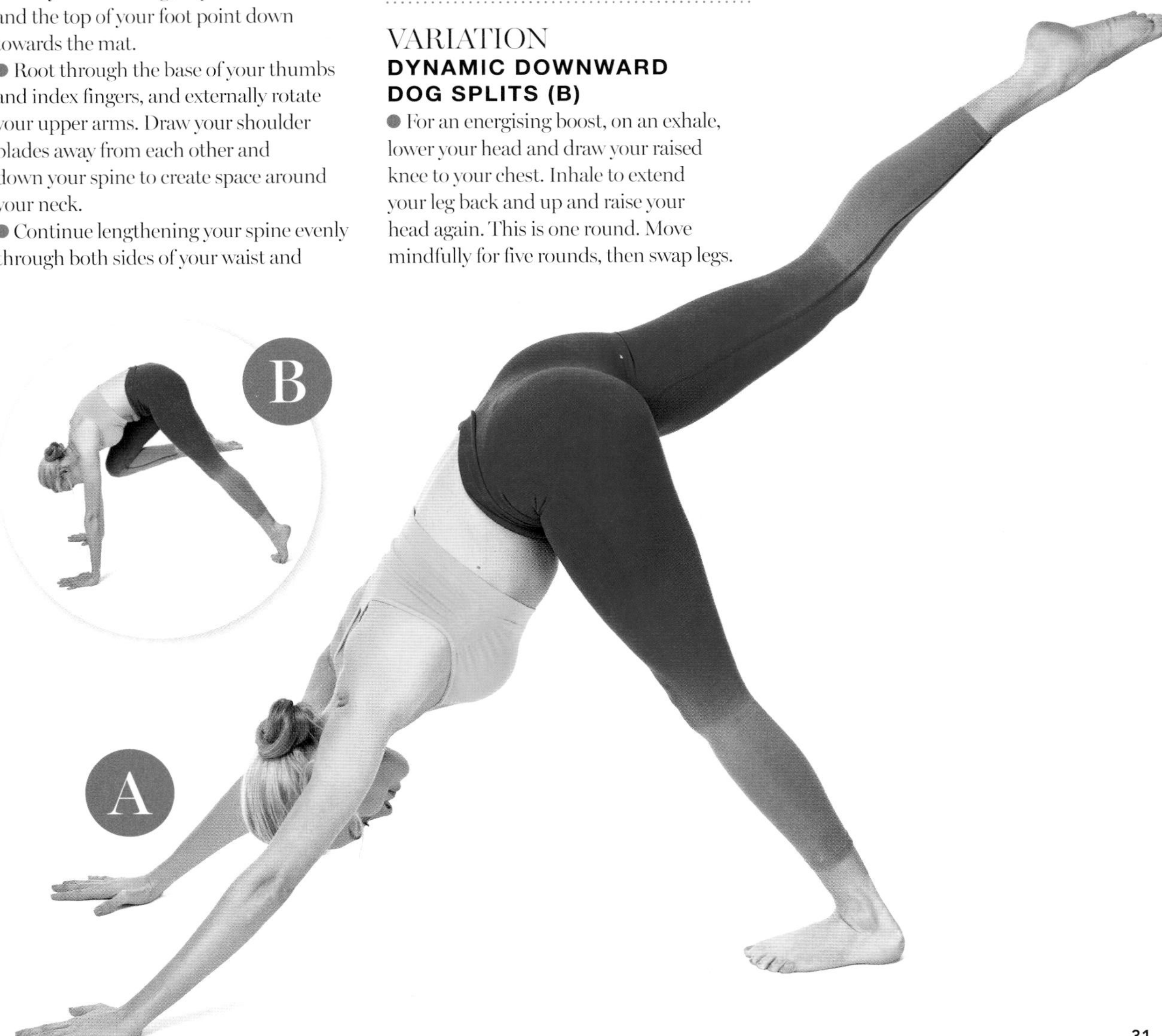

EAGLE POSE
GARUDASANA

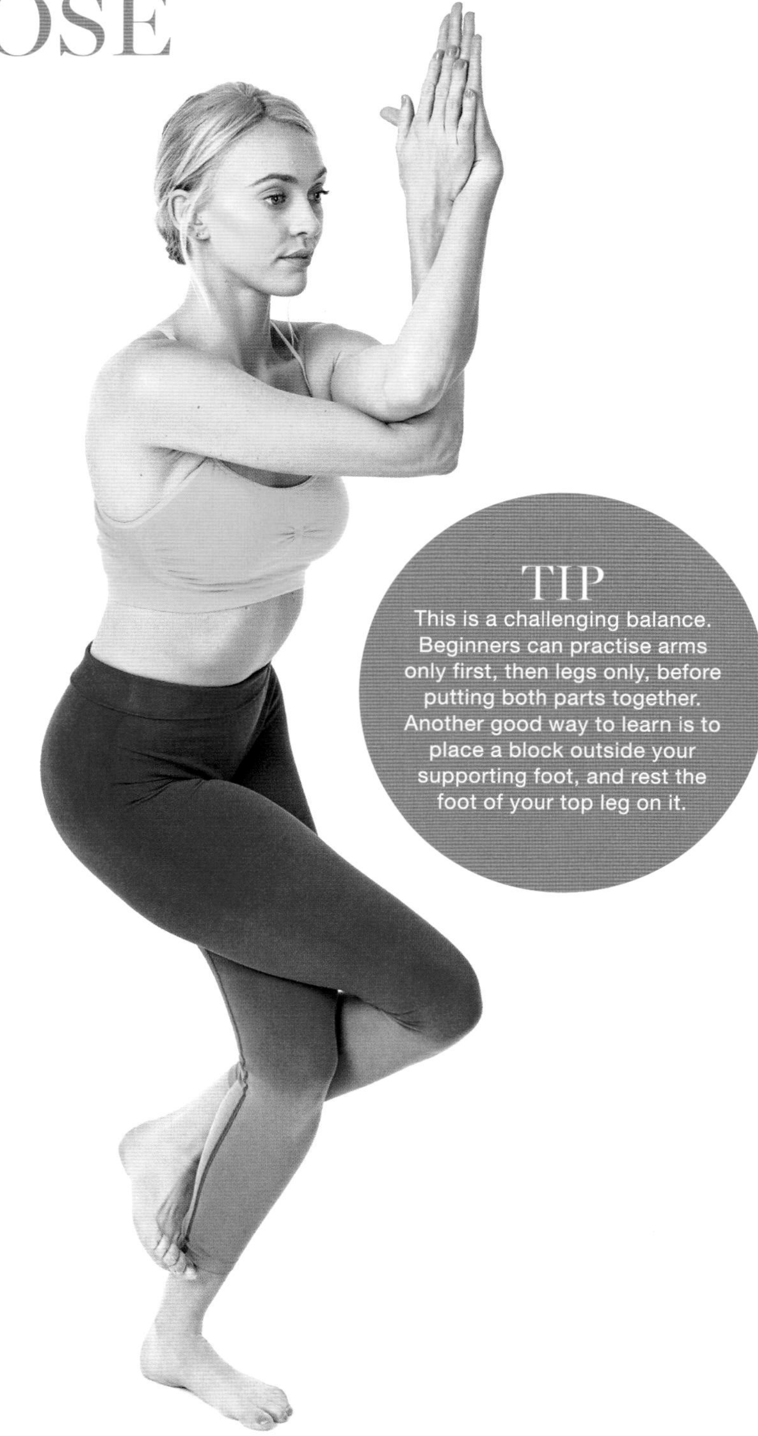

● Stand in Mountain pose (p44) and take a few moments to feel connected to the earth. Lift your toes, spread them wide, then float them back down to the ground. Root through your big and little toes, lift your arches and let the weight of your body sink into your feet. Breathe.

● When you feel grounded, take your weight onto your left foot, bend your left knee and place your right thigh over your left thigh, then wrap your right shin behind your left calf, hooking your toes round. Gaze on a fixed point ahead of you to aid your balance.

● Softly inhale as you float your arms out to the sides to shoulder height. On an exhale, cross your arms in front of you, left elbow on top of right, then intertwine your forearms to bring your palms together (or, for beginners, the backs of your hands), your thumbs facing you and fingertips pointing up.

● With your forearms vertical, draw your shoulder blades down your spine, and raise your elbows to open up the space between your shoulder blades.

● Breathe deeply into your belly to help you stay focused and balanced. Notice if you can keep your mind open and relaxed, despite your body being asymmetrical and twisted.

● Stay in the pose for five deep breaths, then exhale to unfurl your body. Pause in Mountain pose (p44) for a few moments, then repeat on the other side.

GOOD FOR

- Relieves stiff shoulders
- Boosts confidence
- Improves balance
- Aids concentration

TIP

This is a challenging balance. Beginners can practise arms only first, then legs only, before putting both parts together. Another good way to learn is to place a block outside your supporting foot, and rest the foot of your top leg on it.

EASY POSE
SUKHASANA

- Sit on your mat and cross your legs at your shins, so your lower legs are parallel to the front edge of the mat. Use your hands to draw one buttock and then the other away from your mid-line. This will help you root into the ground through your sitting bones.
- Flex your feet to stabilise and protect your knees, then place your hands (or fingertips) either side of your hips, and root down as you draw your navel to your spine and lengthen up out of your pelvis.
- Open your chest, draw your shoulder blades down your back and lift through your crown. Lengthen the back of your neck and softly close your eyes, or gaze a few feet in front of you on the floor.
- Rest your hands on your knees and allow your weight to sink into the floor on each exhale (A). Let your mind become still.
- Breathe calmly and evenly into your abdomen as long as is comfortable, then gently open your eyes.

GOOD FOR
- Grounding and centring
- Soothes your nervous system
- Calms and settles your mind

VARIATIONS
EASY TWIST (B)
- From Easy pose, place your left hand on the floor behind your left buttock, fingers pointing backwards, and rest your right palm on the outside of your left knee. Inhale as you root through your sitting bones to lift your spine out of your pelvis. On an exhale, slowly rotate your spine to the left, moving in a spiral from your waist initially, then your upper body. Inhale, lengthen through the crown of your head, and exhale further into the twist. Draw the kidney area forwards and abdomen towards your navel. Inhale one last time, exhale, release further into the twist, turning your head to look over your left shoulder if comfortable for your neck. Inhale back to centre and repeat on the other side.

EASY SIDE STRETCH (C)
- From Easy pose, inhale and sweep your right arm in an arc overhead. Exhale. On your next inhale, root through your right sitting bone, and lift out of your waist to elongate your right side. As you exhale, draw your right hand further over to the left, taking care to keep your body on the same plane, not leaning forwards or back. Inhale, root down and lengthen a little more, then fold further to the left on an exhale. Take one more deep breath here, inhale back to centre, then lower your arm on an exhale and repeat on the other side.

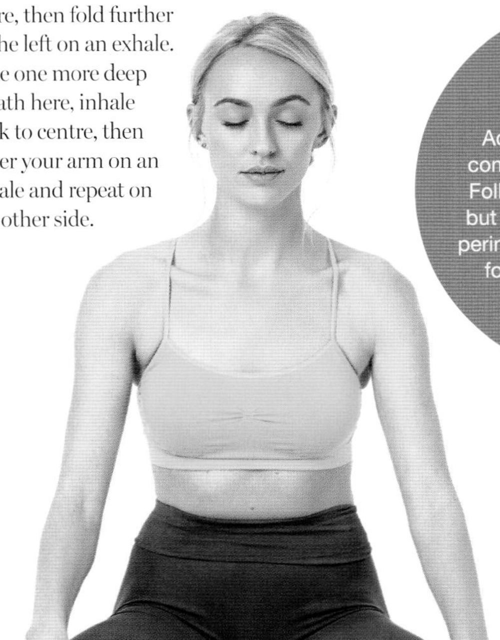

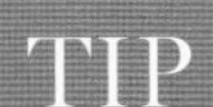

Some people find Accomplished pose more comfortable than Easy pose. Follow the guidelines above, but take your left heel to your perineum and let your left knee fold out to the side. Bring your right foot in and align your heels.

EXTENDED CHILD'S POSE
UTTHITA BALASANA

● Kneeling on your mat, take three breaths into your belly, then draw your knees apart and bring your big toes together, heels wide. Sit back on the soles of your feet and rest your palms on your thighs.
● Inhale as you root into your sitting bones to lengthen your spine. On an exhale, slowly walk your hands forwards, as you lower your torso between your thighs.
● Take your hands shoulder-width apart, palms down, fingers spread and middle fingers pointing forwards. Actively root your hands into the floor, keep your elbows off the mat and draw your arms into your their sockets as you slide your shoulder blades down your back.
● Exhale and lower your head, gently resting your forehead on the floor, a block or a bolster, depending on your flexibility. Softly close your eyes (A).
● Breathe deeply and evenly into your back body for five breaths, sinking deeper into the mat on each exhale. As you extend through to your fingertips, reach your tailbone back to your heels.
● On an exhale, use your hands to gently bring you up to a comfortable seated position. Pause for a moment to register the effects of the pose.

VARIATIONS
CHILD'S POSE (B)
● Take your hands beside your hips, palms facing upwards. Turn your head to rest on one side, remembering to create space around your neck by drawing your shoulders away from your ears. Rest here for up to five minutes, turning your head half-way through.

EXTENDED CHILD'S POSE WITH SIDE STRETCH (C)
● From Extended child's pose, inhale, ground your hands on the mat, raise your head and walk your hands round to your left. On an exhale, release your right hip back onto your right foot. Breathe into your right side body and feel the expansion of your ribs. Take two more breaths here, then exhale to walk your hands back to the centre and repeat on the other side.

GOOD FOR
● Relieves stress and fatigue
● Encourages introspection
● Nurturing
● Calming

TIP
If your spine rounds excessively, come back up to kneeling, place your thumbs in your hip creases (between the top of your thigh and lower abdomen), and push down and backwards. This will help you fold from your hips, rather than your waist.

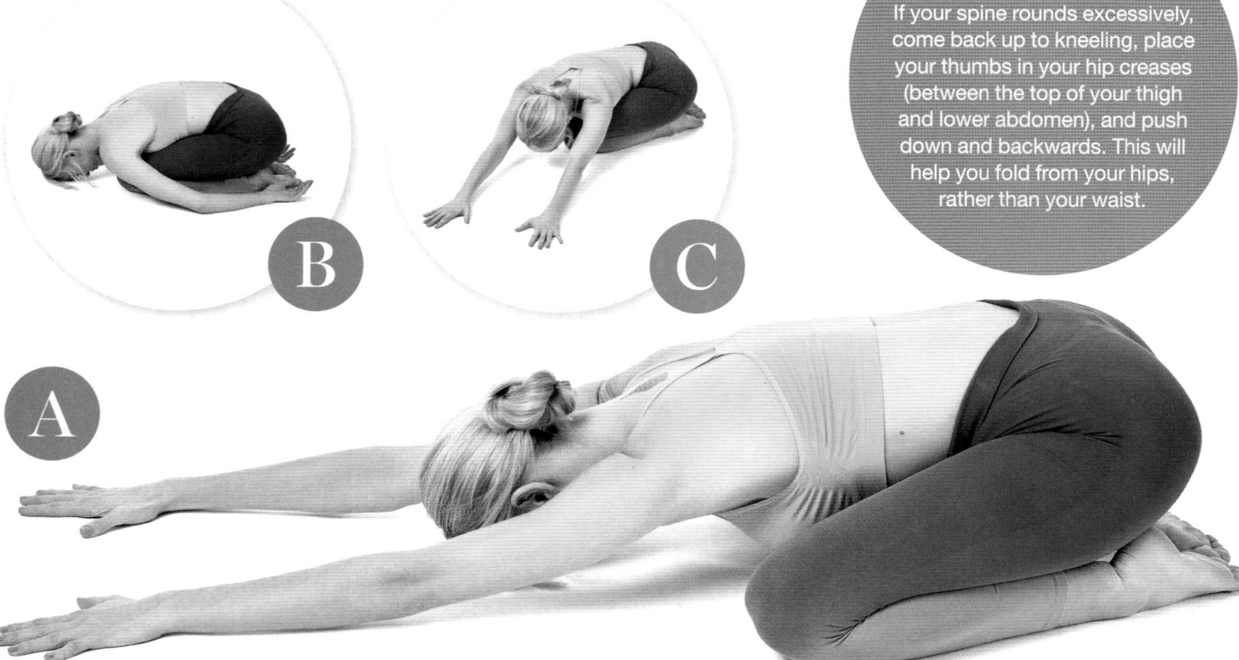

EXTENDED HAND TO TOE POSE

UTTHITA HASTA PADANGUSTHASANA

● From Mountain pose (p44), transfer your weight over your left foot. Spread your toes and ground yourself through the base of your big and little toes. Lift your inner arch.
● Wrap a strap around the ball of your right foot and hold the ends in your right hand, placing your left hand on your left hip.
● Draw your navel to your spine, your shoulders down your spine and lift though the crown. When you feel ready, exhale and extend your right leg out to the side, using the strap as support. Your leg may be bent initially, but over time, you'll be able to straighten it as your balance improves.
● Extend your left arm out to the side and take three to five breaths, directing your energy out through your extended limbs. To come out of the pose, exhale and gently lower your hands and foot. Pause for a moment before repeating on the other side.

GOOD FOR

● Balance
● Strength
● Steadiness
● Focus

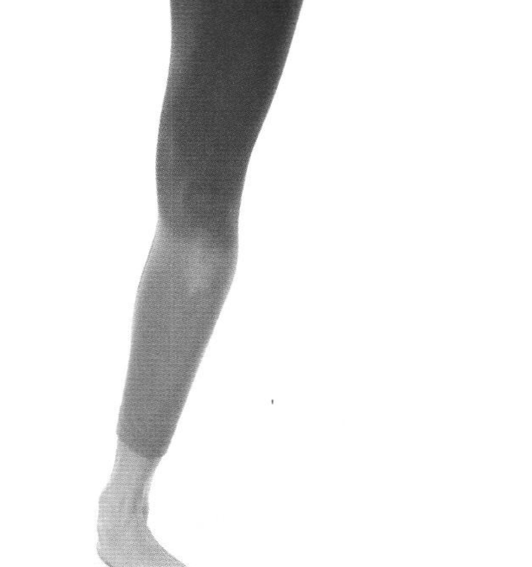

TIP

Gradually shorten the length of the strap as you gain flexibility and strength. Once you feel confident with your balance, do the pose without a strap, resting your extended hand on a wall if you need to.

GARLAND POSE
MALASANA

- Centre yourself in Mountain pose (p44) then, when you feel ready, step your feet wider than hip-width apart. Inhale, and on an exhale, gently crouch down into a low squat, taking your hands to the floor in front of you.
- Turn your feet out, so that your knees are over your toes, then lower your heels, taking your feet as far apart as needed to anchor your heels firmly into the ground.
- Lift your hands into prayer position and let your tailbone release to the mat.
- Press your palms together as you root through your feet, and push your upper arms into your inner thighs, your thighs into your arms. This will help you lift out of your pelvis to lengthen through your spine.
- Draw your shoulder blades down your back and let your chest expand. Take five to 10 deep breaths into your belly.
- When you're ready to come out, release your hands and come to a comfortable seated position for a few breaths while you register the effects of the pose.

GOOD FOR
- Relieves tension in your back
- Loosens your hips
- Calming
- Aids focus

TIP
This can be a strong pose. If your heels don't touch the floor place a folded blanket underneath them to support you.

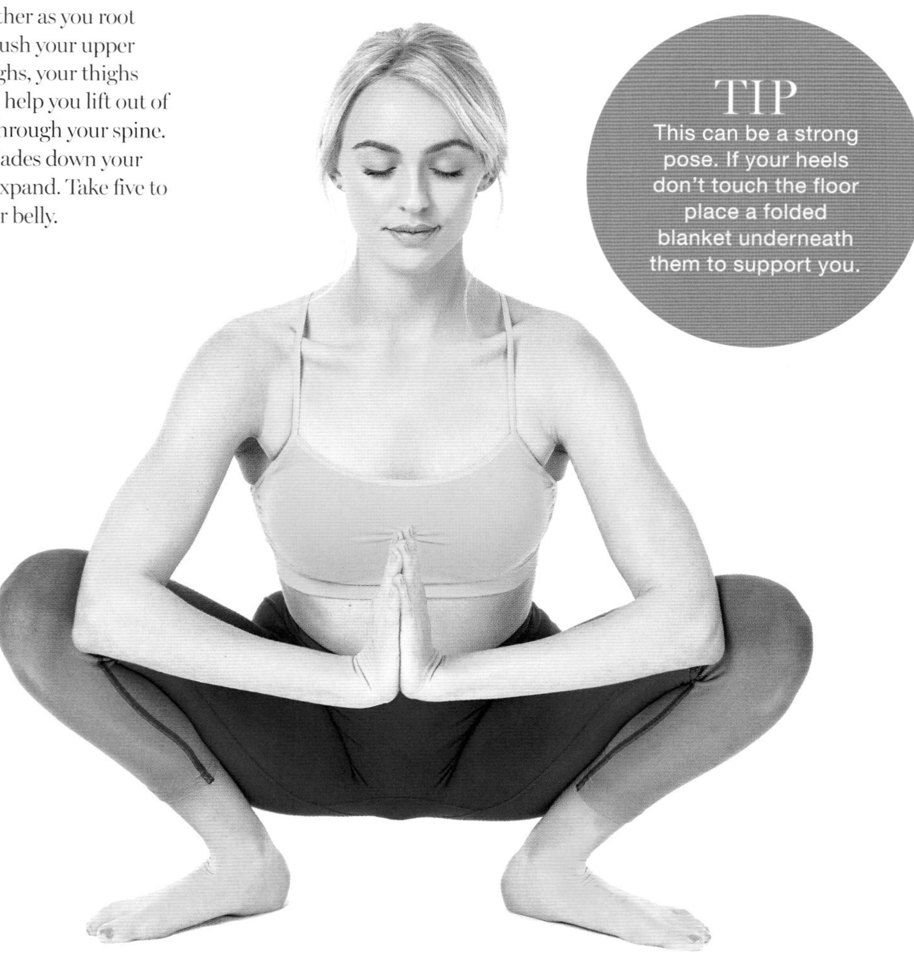

GODDESS POSE
DEVIASANA

● Take a few breaths to become centred in Mountain pose (p44). When you feel ready, step your feet wide apart and turn your toes out 45 degrees. Spread your toes and ground through your big toes and the outer edges of your feet.
● Inhale into your belly. As you exhale, bend your knees over your middle toes, going only as far as will enable you to keep your spine vertical. If your knees fall inwards, bring your toes in slightly or step your feet closer together.
● Lengthen your tailbone towards the floor, and draw your belly button towards your spine.
● Inhale as you circle your arms out to the sides, to shoulder height, then bend your elbows 90 degrees, to take your forearms to vertical. Turn your palms to face forwards (A). Exhale as you sink deeper into the pose.
● Breathe deeply and evenly for five to 10 breaths, feeling the grounded strength of your legs and the gentle opening of your hips and heart.
● When you feel ready to come out of the pose, take your hands to your belly, right over left, and pause for a moment, connecting to your centre. Inhale as you root through your right foot to step your left and then right foot to the centre.

GOOD FOR
● Grounding
● Opens your hips
● Balances masculine and feminine energy: willpower and receptivity
● Strengthens your arms and legs

VARIATION (B)
● For a calming version of Goddess, bring your hands to prayer position and breathe deeply into your belly for five breaths.

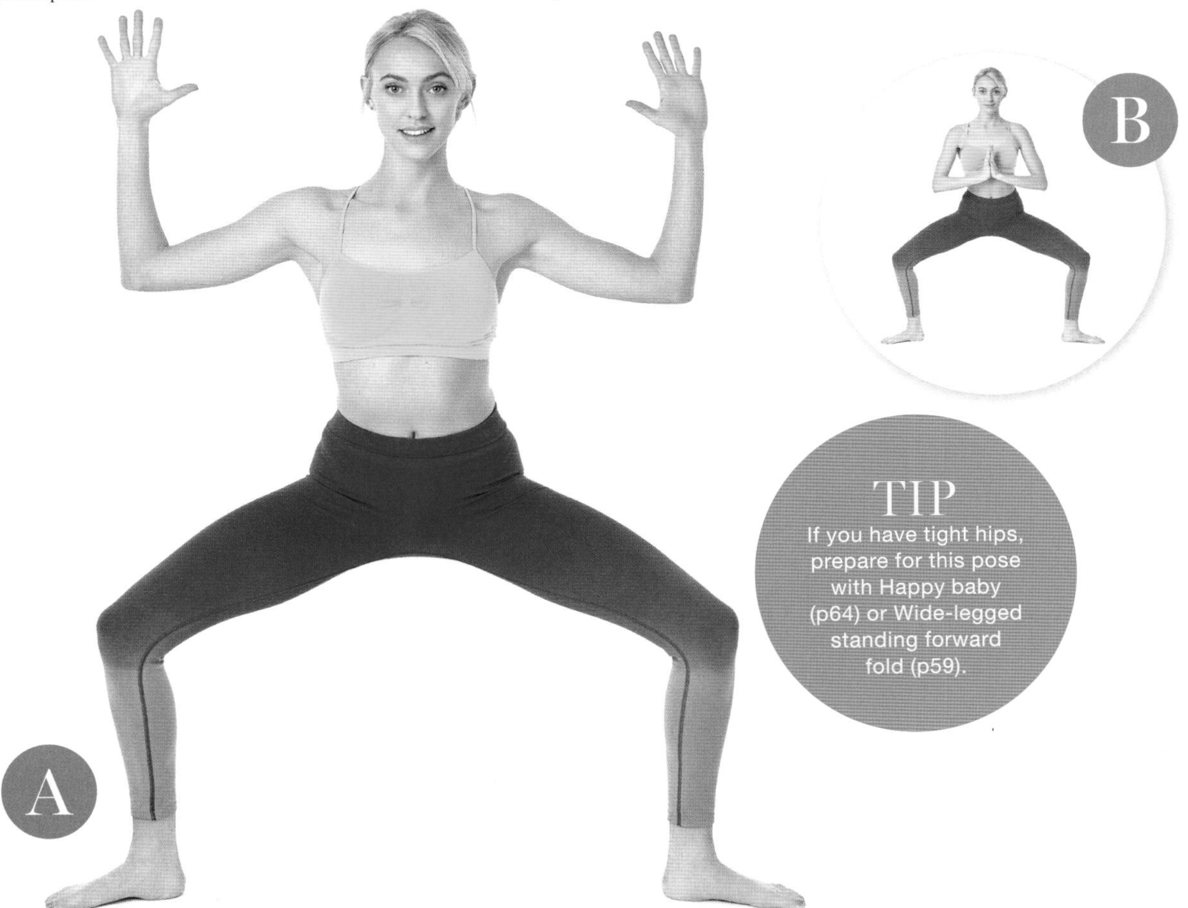

TIP
If you have tight hips, prepare for this pose with Happy baby (p64) or Wide-legged standing forward fold (p59).

HALF MOON
ARDHA CHANDRASANA

- From Triangle pose (p55), to your right, step your back foot in slightly and place your right hand on the floor about a foot in front and slightly outside your right foot.
- Keeping your right leg bent, place your left hand on your left hip and root through your right foot as you lean into the block until your left leg feels 'empty'. Inhale as you float your left leg up to hip height. Flex your ankle, spread your toes and extend through the ball of your left foot.
- Ground your right foot into the floor as you straighten your supporting leg and rotate your chest and pelvis open to the left, so your hips and shoulders are stacked one above the other.
- Keeping a soft gaze towards the floor, inhale and raise your left hand up to the ceiling.
- Breathe evenly from your belly for three to five breaths, imagining there are lines of energy travelling from your centre out through each limb.
- If you are a beginner, you can place your lower hand on a block, remembering to spread your fingertips and root into the ground to lift your torso upwards.
- Exhale to lower your leg, then pause in Wide-legged standing forward fold (p59) before repeating on the other side.

GOOD FOR

- Easing fatigue
- Opening your ribs/improving breathing
- Aiding your balance and focus
- Helps stress and anxiety

TIP

For extra stability in this pose, and to experience the correct alignment, try practising it with your back against a wall. As you progress, rest only your back foot against the wall.

HALF SQUAT
SKANDASANA

● From standing, lower into Crescent (p29) with your right leg back. Take both hands to the inside of your left foot. Walk your hands round to your right as you pivot on the ball of your left foot and heel of your right foot to face the long side of your mat.
● Sit back on your left heel, spreading the toes of your left foot and taking your left knee out to the side. Activate your right foot by pointing your toes to the ceiling. Root down through your left toes as you inhale to lift your torso, shoulder blades sliding down your spine. Bring your hands together into prayer position.
● Continue rooting down to lengthen through your spine, counterbalancing this by drawing your shoulders down your back. Focus on a fixed point ahead to aid your balance and breathe deeply and evenly for three to five breaths (A).
● When ready, lower your hands to the floor, walk them to your right as you transfer your weight onto your right foot, and repeat the pose on the other side.
● To come out, pivot to the right to come into Crescent in the opposite direction, with your hands either side of your front foot, then step your back leg forwards to bring your feet together. Slowly uncurl your spine to return to standing.

GOOD FOR
● Calms your mind
● Aids balance
● Strengthens your legs

VARIATION (B)
● This is a challenging balance. Practise by resting your hands on the floor and gradually raise them into prayer position, increasing the time you spend in prayer as your strength and balance improves.

B

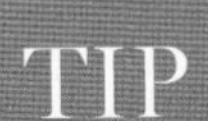

To aid your balance, focus on a point a few feet in front of you.

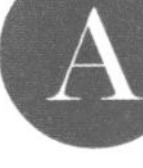

HERO POSE
VIRASANA

● Come onto all fours with your knees slightly apart. Have your shins parallel, tops of your feet flat on the floor and your toes pointing directly backwards.

● Using your hands as a support, gently lower your sitting bones onto your heels, or, if this isn't possible, onto a block or bolster placed lengthwise between your feet. Draw the flesh of your buttocks out to the sides to allow your sitting bones to separate and your tailbone to release towards the floor. If necessary, adjust your pelvis to take it into neutral.

● As your tailbone drops, lift up through your spine, maintaining its vertical alignment as you take your front ribs slightly in towards your back ribs, and separate your collar bones to create space in your chest.

● Draw your shoulder blades down your back and let your head balance evenly and lightly on the top of your spine, lengthening the back of your neck and extending up through the crown.

● Gently close your eyes and rest your hands on your thighs, palms up or down, whichever feels most comfortable (A).

● Breathe fully and deeply in the pose and allow yourself to experience your body as it now is, letting your weight sink deeper on the exhale, a gentle expansion on the inhale. Remain in the pose for up to one minute.

GOOD FOR

- Centring
- Eases high blood pressure
- Promotes healthy knees
- Strengthens the top of your feet

VARIATIONS

HERO WITH BACKBEND (B)

● From Hero pose, take your hands behind your back and rest on your fingertips. Take a couple of breaths to centre yourself, then take a deep breath in as you slightly arch your back to lift your chest. Draw your shoulder blades down your spine and gaze softly ahead. For an extra stretch, raise your buttocks. Take a couple more breaths, then gently lower on an exhale.

HERO TWIST (C)

● From Hero, place your right hand on the floor behind your right buttock, fingers pointing backwards, and rest your left palm on the outside of your right knee. Inhale as you root through your sitting bones to lift your spine out of your pelvis. On an exhale, slowly rotate your spine to the right. On each inhale, lengthen through the crown of your head and exhale further into the twist. Inhale back to centre and repeat on the other side.

TIP
A folded blanket behind your knees will relieve pressure on them. Alternatively, sit on several blocks. If you have tight ankles, place a rolled blanket underneath the front of them for support.
A
B
C

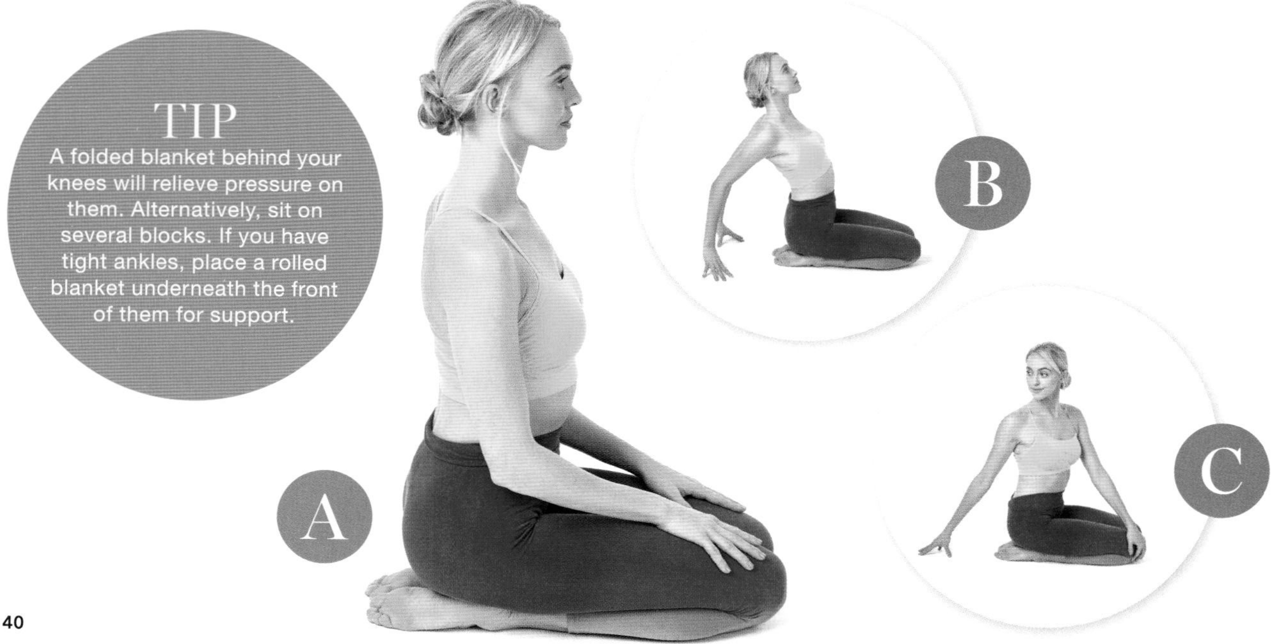

HIGH LUNGE
ALANASANA

● Stand with your feet hip-width apart, inner edges parallel. Take a couple of deep breaths into your belly, allowing your weight to sink towards the earth on the out-breath.
● Fold forwards from your hips and place your hands either side of your feet, resting on your fingertips. Take a large step back with your left leg to rest on the ball of your foot. Straighten your leg and extend through your back heel. Your right knee is directly over your right ankle, aligned with your middle toes.
● Ground through your big and little toes, and raise the inner arch of your right foot.
● With your hands on your hips, take your right hip back and your left hip forwards to square your pelvis, then bring your thighs towards the mid-line.
● Draw your navel towards your spine, then, on an inhale, simultaneously lengthen your spine out of your pelvis as you draw your shoulder blades down your spine.
● On your next inhale, sweep your arms out to the sides and overhead (A).
● Breathe evenly into your belly for five deep breaths, then release your arms on an exhale, step your back foot forwards and repeat on the other side.

GOOD FOR
● Strengthens your legs
● Releases tension in your hips
● Aids balance

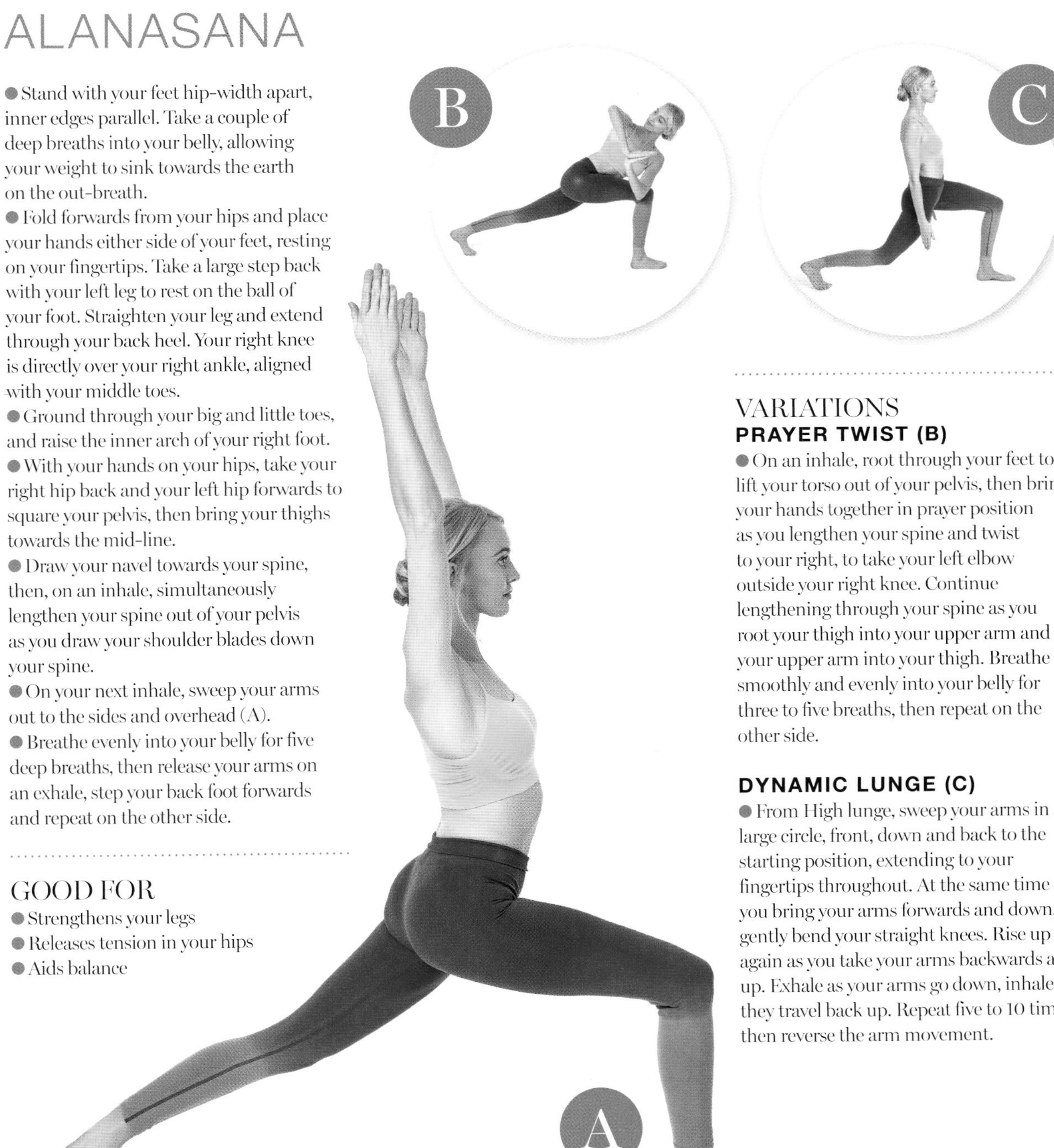

VARIATIONS
PRAYER TWIST (B)
● On an inhale, root through your feet to lift your torso out of your pelvis, then bring your hands together in prayer position as you lengthen your spine and twist to your right, to take your left elbow outside your right knee. Continue lengthening through your spine as you root your thigh into your upper arm and your upper arm into your thigh. Breathe smoothly and evenly into your belly for three to five breaths, then repeat on the other side.

DYNAMIC LUNGE (C)
● From High lunge, sweep your arms in a large circle, front, down and back to the starting position, extending to your fingertips throughout. At the same time as you bring your arms forwards and down, gently bend your straight knees. Rise up again as you take your arms backwards and up. Exhale as your arms go down, inhale as they travel back up. Repeat five to 10 times then reverse the arm movement.

LEGS UP THE WALL

VIPARITA KARANI

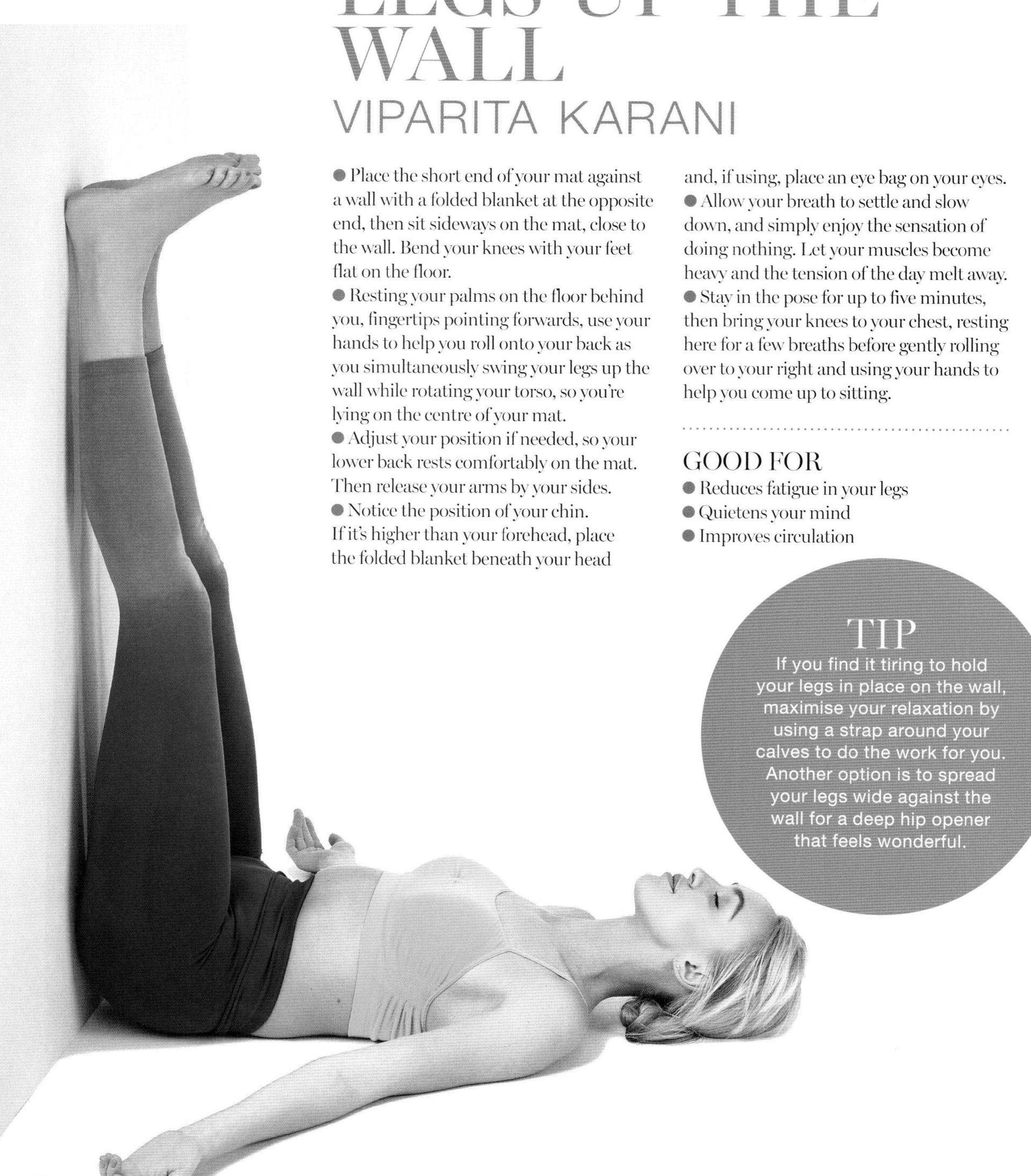

- Place the short end of your mat against a wall with a folded blanket at the opposite end, then sit sideways on the mat, close to the wall. Bend your knees with your feet flat on the floor.
- Resting your palms on the floor behind you, fingertips pointing forwards, use your hands to help you roll onto your back as you simultaneously swing your legs up the wall while rotating your torso, so you're lying on the centre of your mat.
- Adjust your position if needed, so your lower back rests comfortably on the mat. Then release your arms by your sides.
- Notice the position of your chin. If it's higher than your forehead, place the folded blanket beneath your head and, if using, place an eye bag on your eyes.
- Allow your breath to settle and slow down, and simply enjoy the sensation of doing nothing. Let your muscles become heavy and the tension of the day melt away.
- Stay in the pose for up to five minutes, then bring your knees to your chest, resting here for a few breaths before gently rolling over to your right and using your hands to help you come up to sitting.

GOOD FOR

- Reduces fatigue in your legs
- Quietens your mind
- Improves circulation

TIP

If you find it tiring to hold your legs in place on the wall, maximise your relaxation by using a strap around your calves to do the work for you. Another option is to spread your legs wide against the wall for a deep hip opener that feels wonderful.

LIZARD POSE
UTTHAN PRISTHASANA

- From Downward dog (p30), step your right foot forwards between your hands. Raise your right hand as you move the heel/toe of your foot towards the edge of your mat, then lower again. Tuck your back toes under.
- Check that your right knee is directly above your ankle, hug it into the mid-line and ground through the base of your big and little toes.
- Walk your hands slightly forwards as you release your hips forwards and down, and extend your heart forwards to lengthen your spine while simultaneously drawing your shoulders down your back. Lightly draw your navel to your spine (A).
- If comfortable, rest your forearms on the ground (B) or on a block, and remain in the pose for five deep breaths. Then press your hands into the mat to come up and back into Extended child's pose (p34), then repeat on the other side.
- For a gentler pose, try Dragon (p76), lowering your back knee to the ground.

GOOD FOR

- Opens your hips and groin
- Releases tight hip flexors
- Strengthens the inner thigh of your front leg

TIP
This is a strong hip opener, so take it gently and breathe into any areas of discomfort.

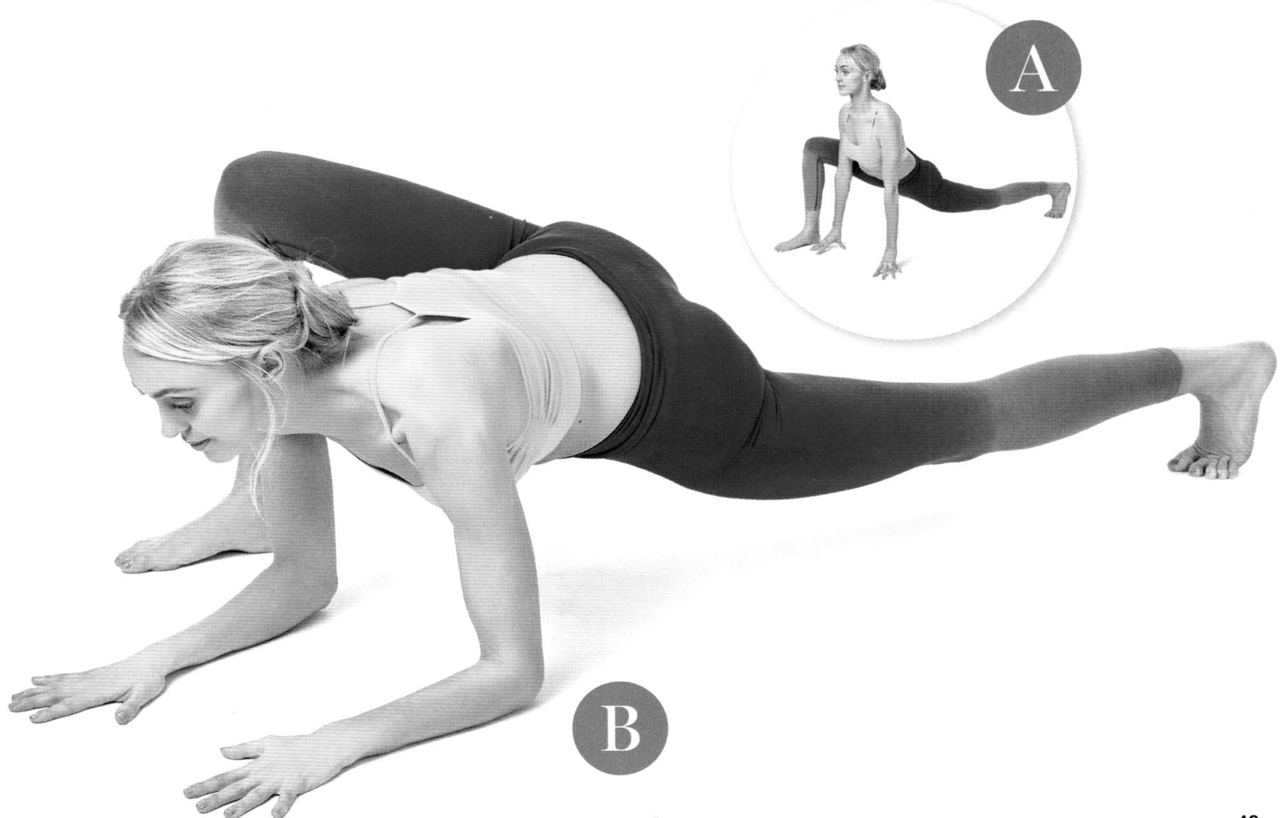

MOUNTAIN POSE
TADASANA

● With your feet together or shoulder-width apart and inner edges parallel, balance your weight evenly between each foot. Spread your toes and root through the base of your big and little toes. Draw your ankles away from each other to lift your inner arches.

● Check that your knees are above your ankles and your pelvis is over your knees. Release your tail and sitting bones so your pelvis is in neutral.

● Draw your navel towards your spine and release your shoulders back and down your spine. Let your arms fall naturally to your sides and allow them to extend gently through to your fingertips.

● Lengthen the back of your neck and soften your throat. Let go of any tension in your jaw and let your gaze be soft.

● As you inhale, lengthen through your crown and as you exhale, maintaining the sense of lift, allow your weight to sink to the floor, and any physical tension in your body to release (A). Stay here for five to 10 deep, slow breaths.

GOOD FOR

● Balance
● Grounding
● Stilling your mind
● Posture

VARIATIONS

PRAYER HANDS (B)

● Bring your hands to your heart, elbows down, palms together and fingertips pointing upwards. Softly, but actively, press each palm into the other. Release and lengthen the back of your neck.

EXTENDED MOUNTAIN (C)

● On a slow, deep inhale, root though your feet as you lift your waist out of your hips to lengthen your spine. At the same time, turn your palms outwards and extend your arms to the sides and overhead to come into Extended mountain pose. On each inhale, root down to lift through your crown, and on each exhale, visualise your breath travelling down your body and out through your feet.

EXTENDED MOUNTAIN SIDE STRETCH (D)

● From Extended mountain pose, ground through your feet as you inhale and lengthen your spine, then exhale and gently draw your arms over to your right to open your left side body. Allow your left hip to move out to the side, bending your right knee a little if this feels more comfortable. Rest in the pose for three to five breaths, then inhale back to centre and repeat on the other side. Exhale to lower your arms.

TIP

At least once, practise this pose with your back against a wall, so you get a sense of how it feels to stand completely straight.

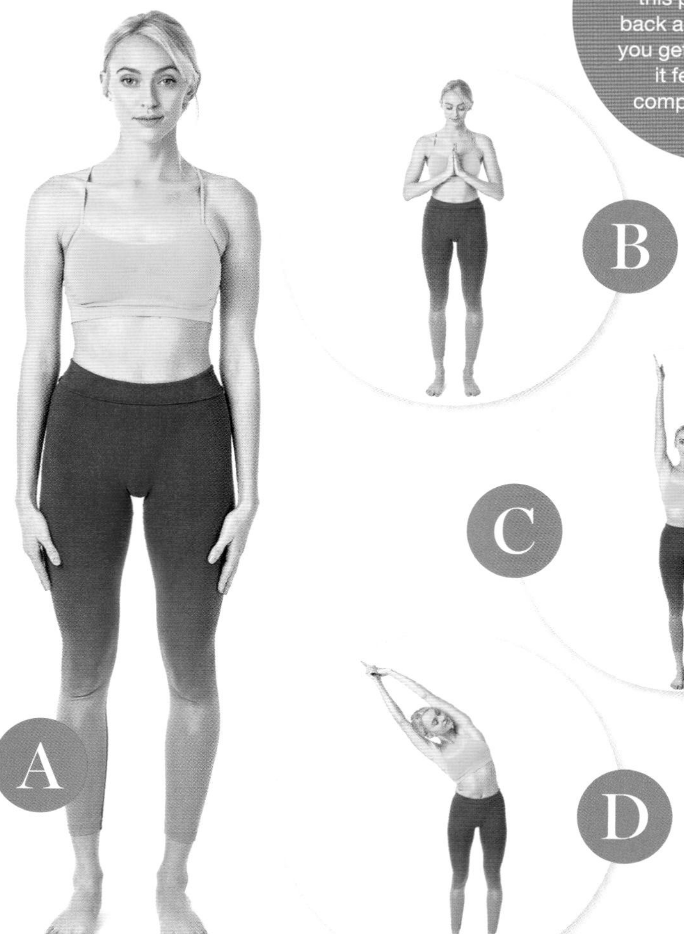

NECTAR OF THE FLOWING MOON

SOMACHANDRASANA

- Close your eyes and take two or three deep breaths into your belly to quieten your mind. Step into a lunge, with your right foot forwards and your hands either side of this foot.
- Inhale, then, on an exhale, take your weight onto your left hand as you pivot clockwise on your front heel, turning your right foot out 90 degrees.
- At the same time, pivot clockwise on your back toes, taking your heel to the left, so you rest on the outer edge of your back foot, sole facing the back of the mat.
- Grounding through your left hand, inhale and arc your right arm forwards and alongside your ear (A). If comfortable for your neck, look up towards your raised hand, otherwise keep your gaze to the floor, and, keeping your legs active, use the contact of your left foot on the mat to lift your chest and lengthen the right side of your body, from your foot to your fingertips.
- On your next exhale, sweep your right arm alongside your top hip, fingertips pointing towards your back foot. Take your gaze towards your left toes or the floor (B).
- Continue moving between these two poses for a few rounds, arcing a little deeper into a backbend on each inhale, softening as your exhale. When you feel ready, exhale to lower, then rest in Child's pose (p34), before repeating on the other side.

GOOD FOR

- Mildly energising
- Opens your heart
- Calming
- Grounding

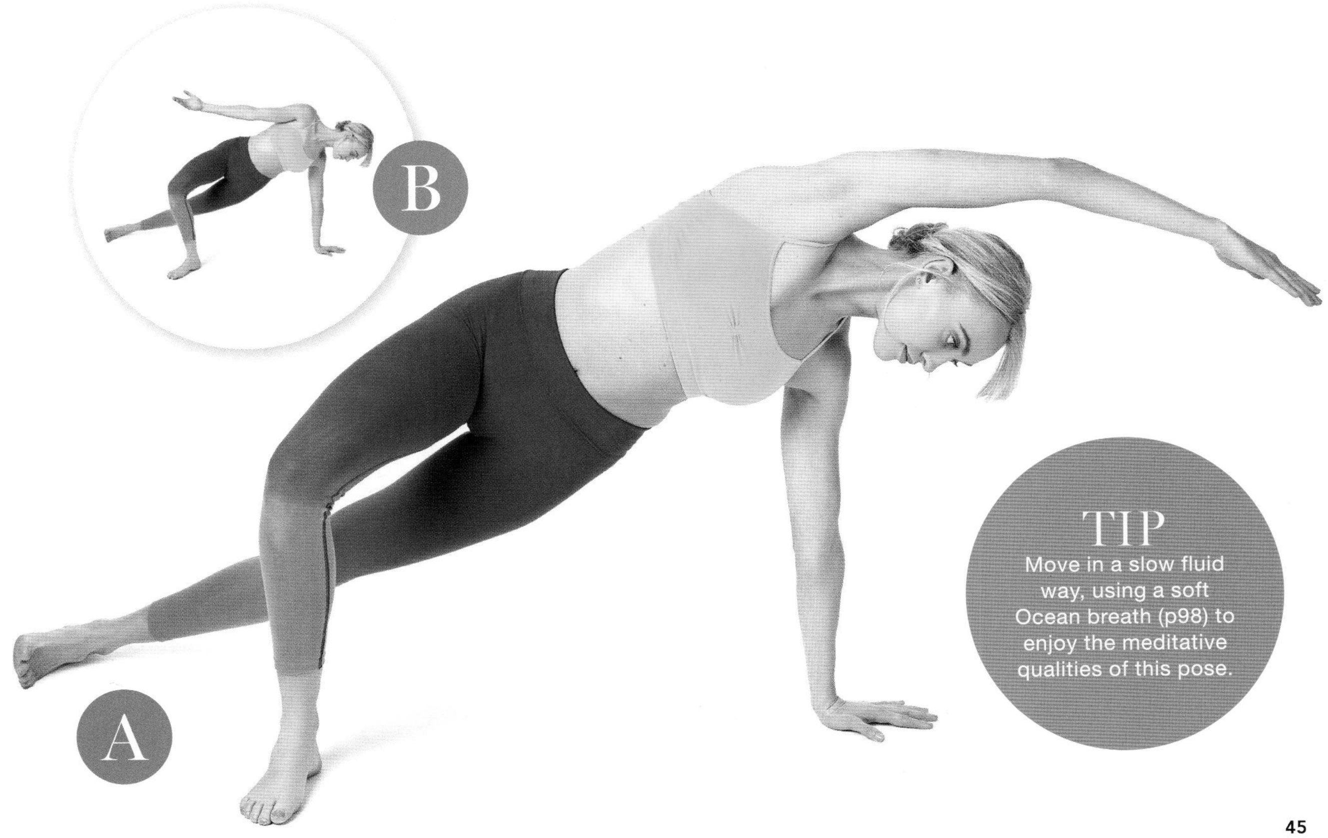

TIP

Move in a slow fluid way, using a soft Ocean breath (p98) to enjoy the meditative qualities of this pose.

PLANK
KUMBHAKASANA

● Start on all fours with your hands shoulder-width apart, directly beneath your shoulders. Spread your fingers, root through the base of your thumb and index finger and straighten your elbows without locking them.

● Step your feet back, resting on the balls of your feet, and straighten your legs to create a diagonal line from your heels to your crown. Tuck in your chin to maintain length in the back of your neck.

● Draw your navel to your spine and spread your shoulder blades apart (A).

● Breathe evenly for five to 10 breaths, then gently lower yourself to the floor on an exhale.

GOOD FOR

- Strengthens your core
- Tones your bottom
- Strengthens your upper body
- Builds focus and stamina

VARIATION
SIDE PLANK (B)

● From Plank, press your right hand into the floor and roll onto the outside edge of your right foot, stacking your body so your left foot is on top of your right, and left knee, hip and shoulder are on top of your right. Draw your navel to your spine and adjust the left side of your body so it doesn't collapse as you inhale, and raise your left arm to the ceiling. If need be, bend your top knee and rest your foot behind the knee of your straight leg.

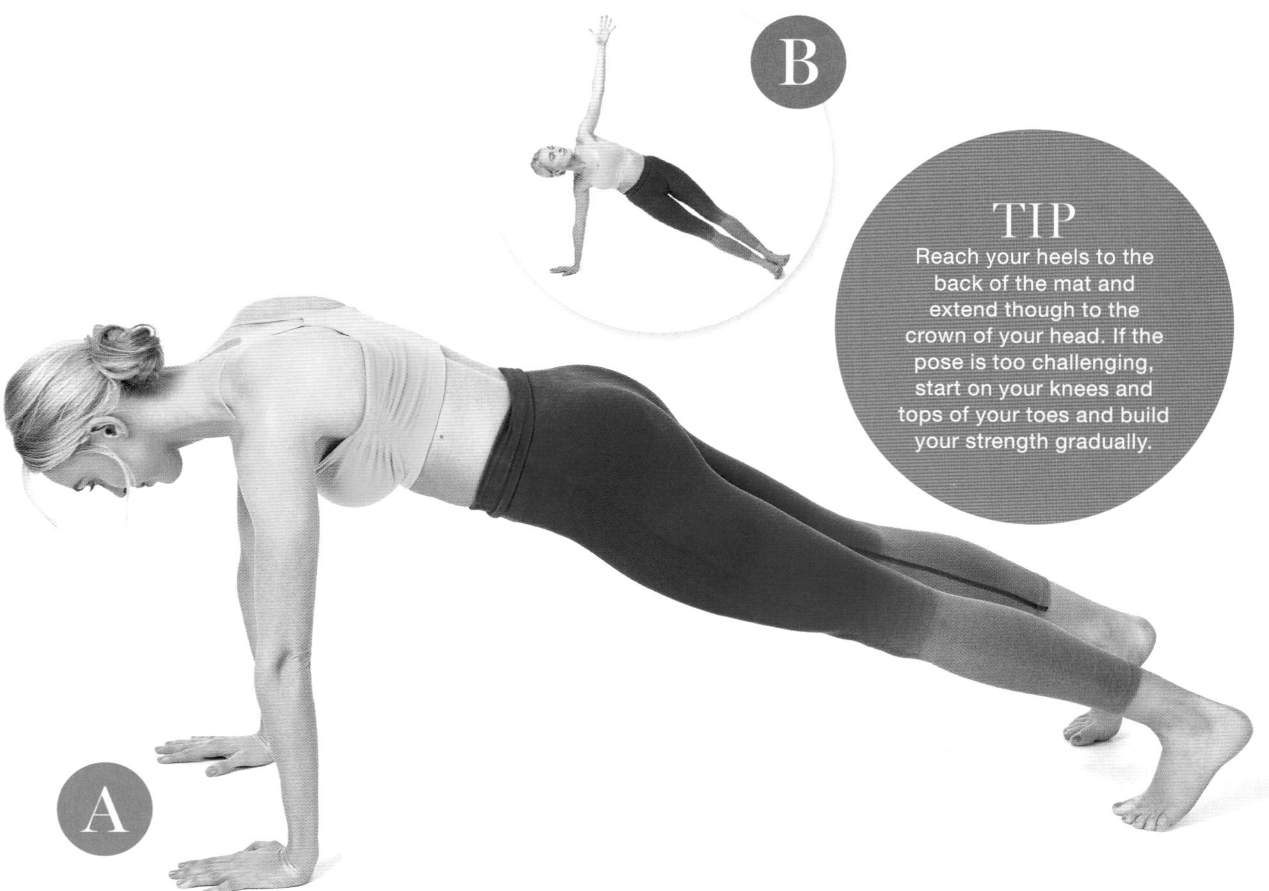

TIP

Reach your heels to the back of the mat and extend though to the crown of your head. If the pose is too challenging, start on your knees and tops of your toes and build your strength gradually.

PYRAMID

PARSVOTTANASANA

- With your feet parallel and hip-width apart, take a large step back with your left leg. Keeping your right foot as it is, pivot on your left heel so your foot is at a 45-degree angle. Spread your toes and root through your right big toe and the outer edge of your left foot. Lift your inner arches by drawing your ankles apart.
- With your hands on your hips, bring your left hip forwards and your right hip back, so your pelvis is facing the front of your mat. Draw your inner thighs towards each other to stabilise the pose.
- Inhale and root down to the ground as you lengthen your spine then, on an exhale, begin to fold forwards, keeping your spine flat. Travel slowly and mindfully until you reach the end of your out-breath, then pause.
- On your next inhale, extend and lengthen your entire spine, then gently release on an exhale to fold further forwards, letting your back naturally curve as you get lower. Continue lengthening and lowering in this way as far as is comfortable, taking your hands to your lower legs or the floor (A).
- Rest in the pose for five to 10 breaths, breathing evenly through your nose. When you feel ready, root through your feet and inhale to return to standing, then exhale to step your feet together. Pause for a moment, then repeat on the other side.
- Beginners, place a block either side of your front foot (B) and work on keeping your hips square to the front of your mat, and lowering to horizontal with a flat back.

GOOD FOR

- Increases blood flow to your head
- Calms your mind
- Aids deep breathing
- Develops balance

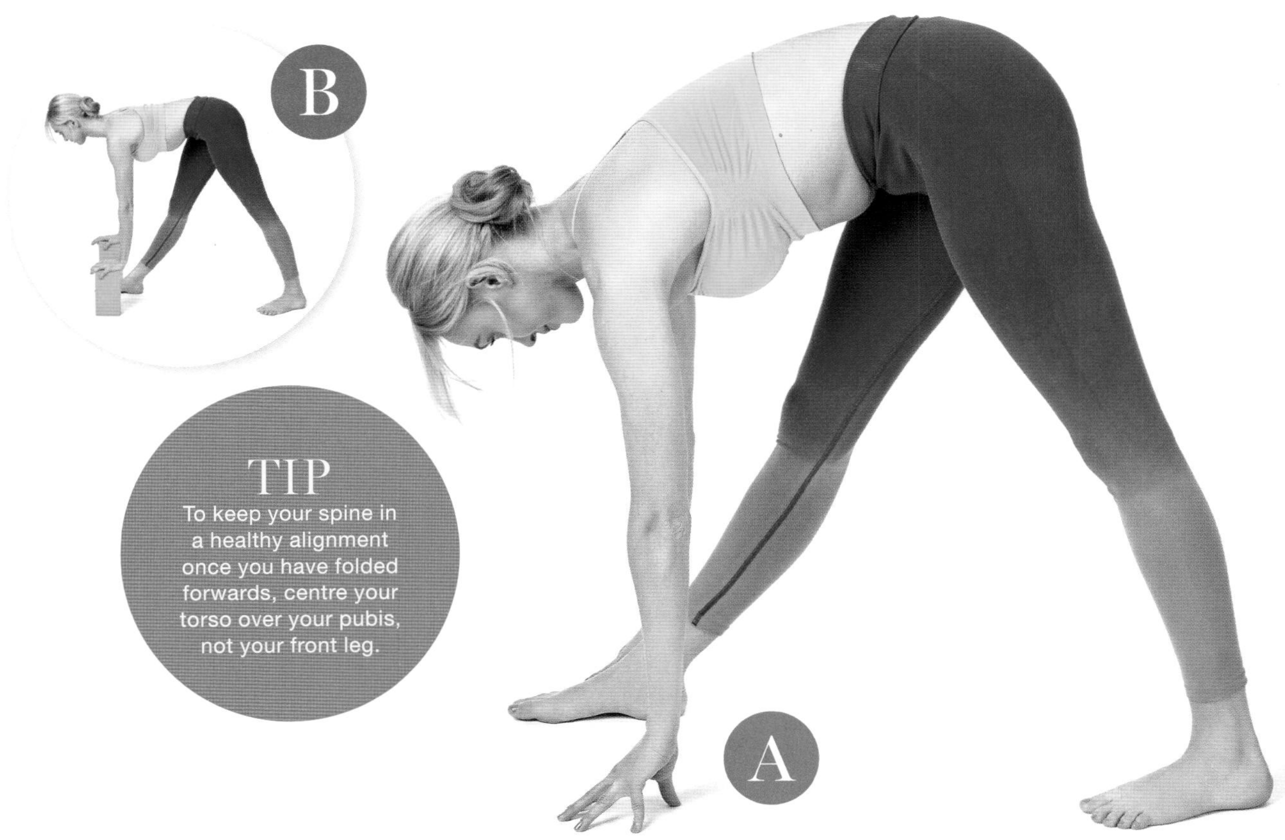

TIP

To keep your spine in a healthy alignment once you have folded forwards, centre your torso over your pubis, not your front leg.

RECLINING TWIST
SUPTA PARIVARTANASANA

- Lie on your back and take a few moments to centre yourself, allowing your breath to deepen and your heartbeat to become slower.
- Hug both knees to your chest, using your forearms to bring your knees in close and draw your shoulder blades down your back. Take a few breaths here, then extend your right leg to the floor, allowing your right thigh to release down to the mat.
- Rest your right hand on your left knee and, on an exhale, guide it over to the right. Extend your left arm to the side, palm facing upwards and, if comfortable, gently turn your head to look to the left.
- Breathe deeply into your left side, enjoying the stretch for 10 deep breaths, then slowly inhale back to centre and repeat on the other side.

GOOD FOR

- Reduces stress
- Releases tension in your spine
- Opens your chest
- Eases stiffness in your lower back

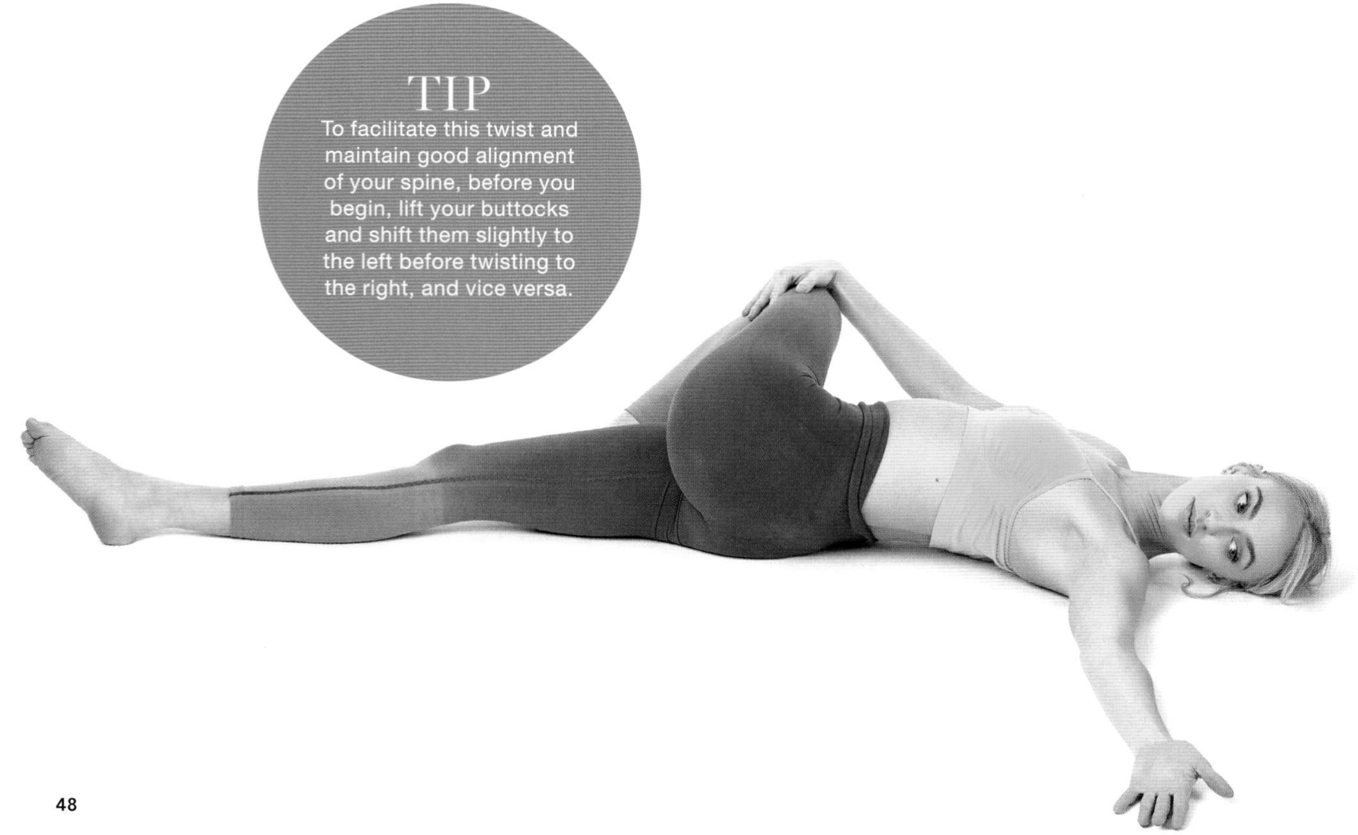

TIP

To facilitate this twist and maintain good alignment of your spine, before you begin, lift your buttocks and shift them slightly to the left before twisting to the right, and vice versa.

RELAXATION POSE

SAVASANA

- Sit on the floor with your knees bent, your feet on the floor and hands resting behind you. Raise your buttocks, and tilt your tailbone forwards to flatten your lower back, then gently release your sacrum to the floor.
- Lower onto your elbows to lie flat on your back and extend your arms a comfortable distance from your sides, palms facing upwards. Extend one leg at a time, taking your feet a little wider than hip-distance apart, and allow your feet to roll out to the sides.
- Wriggle your torso a little, to snuggle your body into the floor then, checking that your arms and legs are symmetrical, rest your head on the centre of the back of your skull. Gently close your eyes.
- Begin to allow any tension in your body to seep away into the floor, consciously letting go on each exhalation.
- Breathe softly and evenly into your belly, letting your eyelids be heavy, and your eyes sink deeper into their sockets. Relax your temples and soften your jaw. Release your neck, shoulders and arms. Invite your belly to expand and your thighs, calves and ankles to relax. Let everything be soft and heavy.
- Allow your muscles to melt into your bones and your bones to sink into the mat.
- Rest for five to 10 minutes. Breathe naturally, allowing your body to experience a sense of expansion as you inhale, and a feeling of softening as you exhale.
- To come out of the pose, without disturbing the atmosphere you've created, slowly wriggle your fingers and toes to bring movement back to your body. Softly slide your arms out to the sides and overhead, and gently stretch your body from your feet to your fingertips. Slowly bring your knees to your chest, wrap your arms around them and gently rock from side to side.
- Roll over to your right side and rest for few moments, then use your left hand to help you come up to sitting.
- Rest in Easy pose (p33) for a minute or two, to acclimatise your spine to being upright once more.
- When you get up, move softly and mindfully, to keep the sense of relaxation with you as you move into the next phase of your day.

GOOD FOR

- Deeply relaxing
- Balances mind, body and spirit
- Rejuvenating
- Reduces fatigue
- Teaches you to be tension free
- Calms your mind

TIP

Be aware of any physical sensations in your body, and if you feel any discomfort, pain or tension, direct your breath into that area and allow the sensation to soften and release as you exhale. Lengthening each out-breath will activate your rest and digest response, deepening the sense of relaxation that you feel.

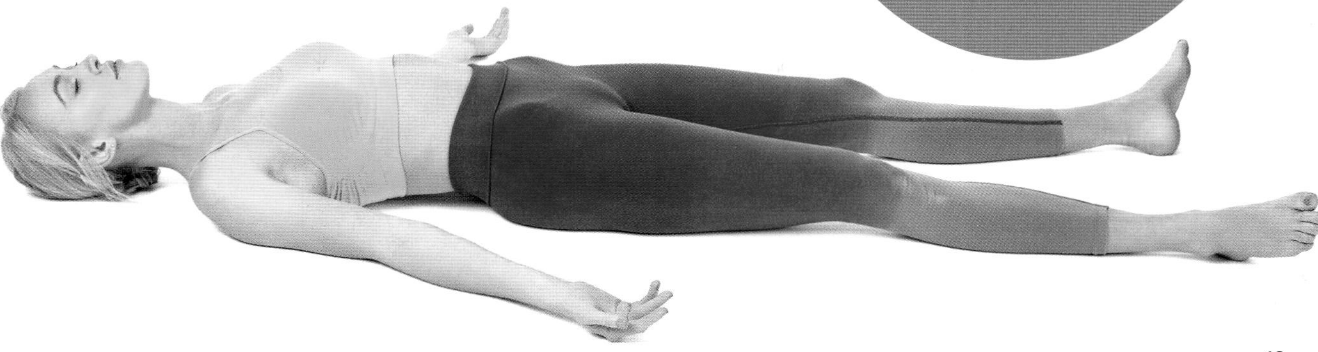

SEATED FORWARD FOLD
PASCHIMOTTANASANA

- Sit with your legs straight out in front of you, feet together, ankles flexed and toes pointing to the ceiling. Extend through the balls of your feet, spread your toes and reach through the base of your big and little toes. Lift your arches and draw the outside edges of your feet slightly towards your body.
- Inhale and take your arms overhead. Exhale as you release your shoulder blades down your back and draw your arms into your shoulder sockets.
- On the next inhalation, root through your sitting bones to extend your spine up out of your pelvis. As you exhale, fold forwards slightly from your hips with a flat back. Pause, then inhale again as you lengthen your spine and, leading from your heart, fold further forwards.
- Continue moving, breath-by-breath, lengthening your front and back spine evenly, as you reach your torso up and forwards to fold over your thighs. As you become lower, release your spine and take your hands to your shins, outer edges of your feet, or clasp your hands behind your feet.
- Maintain the space around your neck by drawing your shoulders away from your ears, and keep your neck long by extending through your crown and drawing your chin to your chest.
- Breathe deeply and evenly in the pose, feeling the strength of your legs and the expansion in your back body as your spine gently undulates with each in- and out-breath.
- When you feel ready, take a deep inhalation and reach up with your crown as you lead with your heart to return to sitting. Rest for a moment or two with your eyes closed as you allow your body to register the effect of the pose.

GOOD FOR

- Rests your mind
- Relieves stress and anxiety
- Reduces fatigue
- Eases insomnia

TIP

If you have tight hamstrings, sit on a folded blanket, bend your knees or use a strap around the balls of your feet. If your back rounds, sitting on a bolster can be helpful.

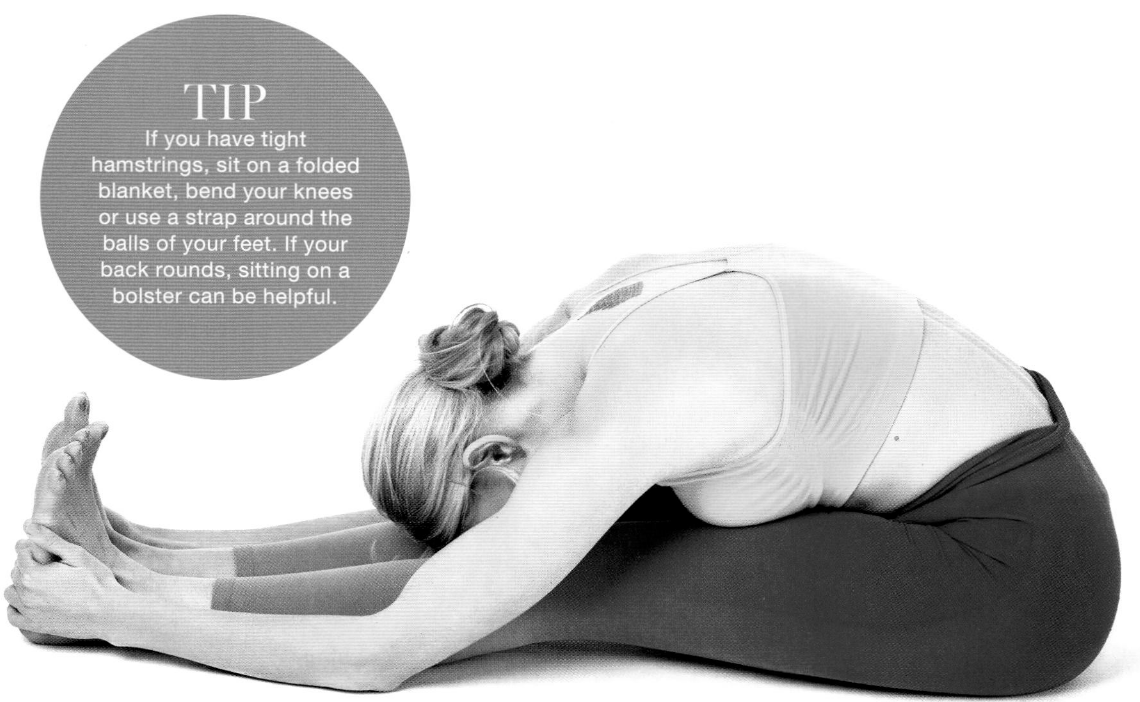

SPONTANEOUS FLOWING HALF SQUAT

SAHAJA ARDHA MALASANA

● Take a moment in Mountain pose (p44) to still your mind. When you feel ready to begin, take your feet wide apart.
● With a smooth flowing breath, allow your upper body to cascade downwards as you slowly transfer your weight to your left foot. At the same time, release your arms and allow them to drape over the floor towards your left foot (A).
● Transfer your weight back to your right, trailing your arms behind you (B).
● Keep your spine long, release your neck and let your upper body and arms move in a flowing, sweeping motion, like seaweed in the ocean as you alternate a few times between your right and left sides, breathing freely. Once you become familiar with the movement, experiment with bending alternate knees as you flow from side to side, bending your right knee as you flow to the right, your left knee as you flow to the left.
● Finish on your right, and pivot in a clockwise direction to come into Lunge, then lower your left knee, and step your right foot back to come into Child's pose (p34). Rest here for a few breaths to absorb the experience of the flowing sequence.

GOOD FOR

● Deeply relaxing
● Frees your neck and spine
● Releases tension in your hips
● Strengthens your legs

TIP

Let your arms flow freely, and allow yourself to express through movement what you need in the moment, maybe tracing featherlight fingertips across the mat, or making large expansive circles as you sway from side to side. Allow your torso to fold over your bent leg to release any tension in your spine.

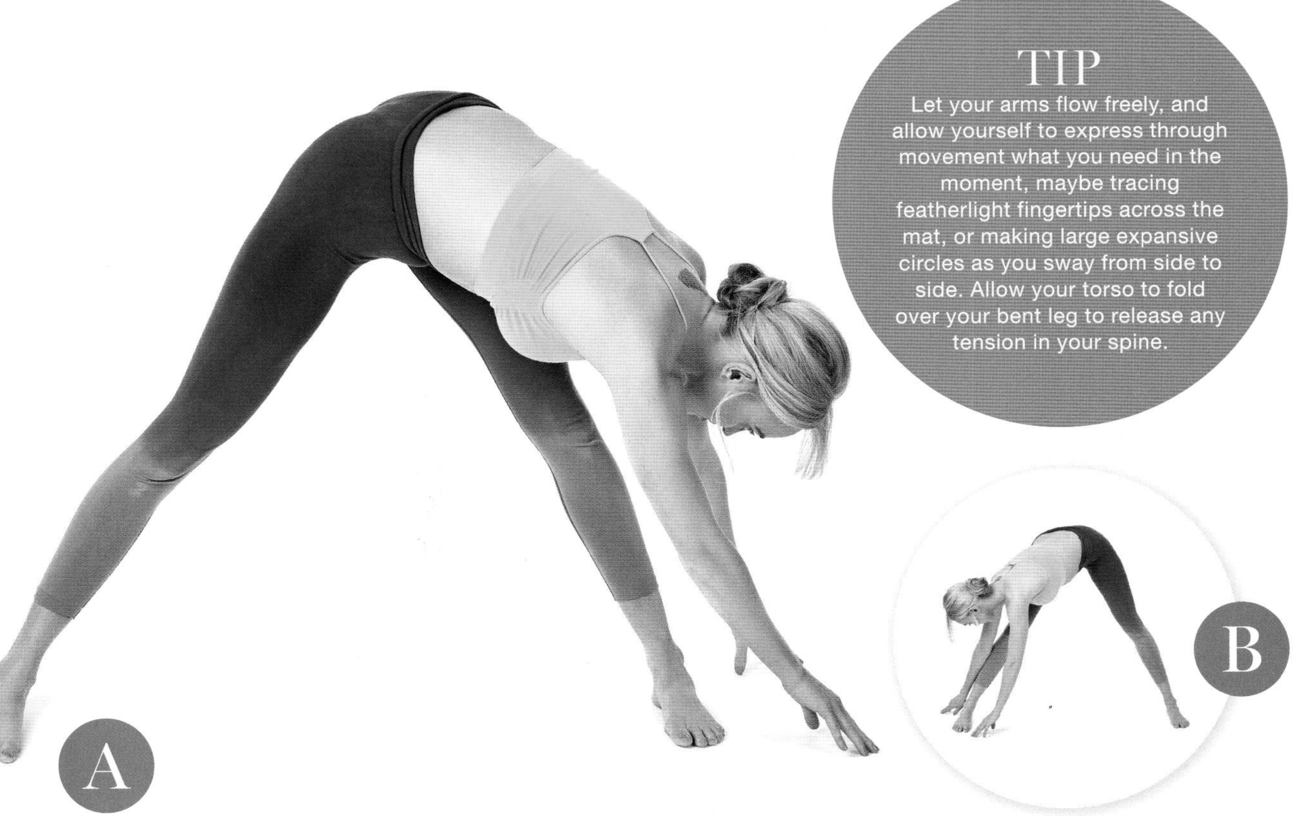

STANDING FORWARD FOLD

UTTANASANA

● From Mountain pose (p44), with your feet hip-distance apart, take your hands to your hips and, on an inhale, root through your feet to lengthen your torso away from your pelvis.

● Exhale, bend your knees slightly and fold forwards from your hips with a flat back. When your spine is parallel to the floor, let your pelvis come into neutral.

● Keeping your knees bent, inhale to lengthen your spine, then, as you exhale, continue folding and allow your chest to rest on your thighs. Release your arms and lay your hands on your shins, ankles or the floor.

● If it feels comfortable, straighten your legs, keeping a microbend in your knees, then allow your upper body to relax fully. Take your tailbone towards the ceiling, and your head closer to the floor (A).

● On each in-breath, feel your spine lengthening and on each out-breath, fold a little deeper.

● Consciously surrender, breathing softly and evenly for several breaths, then inhale to gently uncurl to return to standing.

GOOD FOR

● Calms your nervous system
● Relieves fatigue
● Reduces insomnia
● Regulates your blood pressure

VARIATIONS

HALF STANDING FORWARD FOLD (B)

● From Standing forward fold, knees bent or straight, place your hands a few inches in front of your feet. Inhale as you lengthen your crown away from your tailbone to come up to a flat back. Root through your hands and feet and draw your shoulder blades down your spine. Take five deep breaths and release back into Standing forward fold.

LUNAR FORWARD FOLD (C)

● This soft forward fold is used in the Moon salutation II (p110). Bend your knees and let your torso drape over your thighs. Release your neck and rest the backs of your hands on the floor. Allow your breath to find its natural rhythm, slowing down as your body surrenders to the ground.

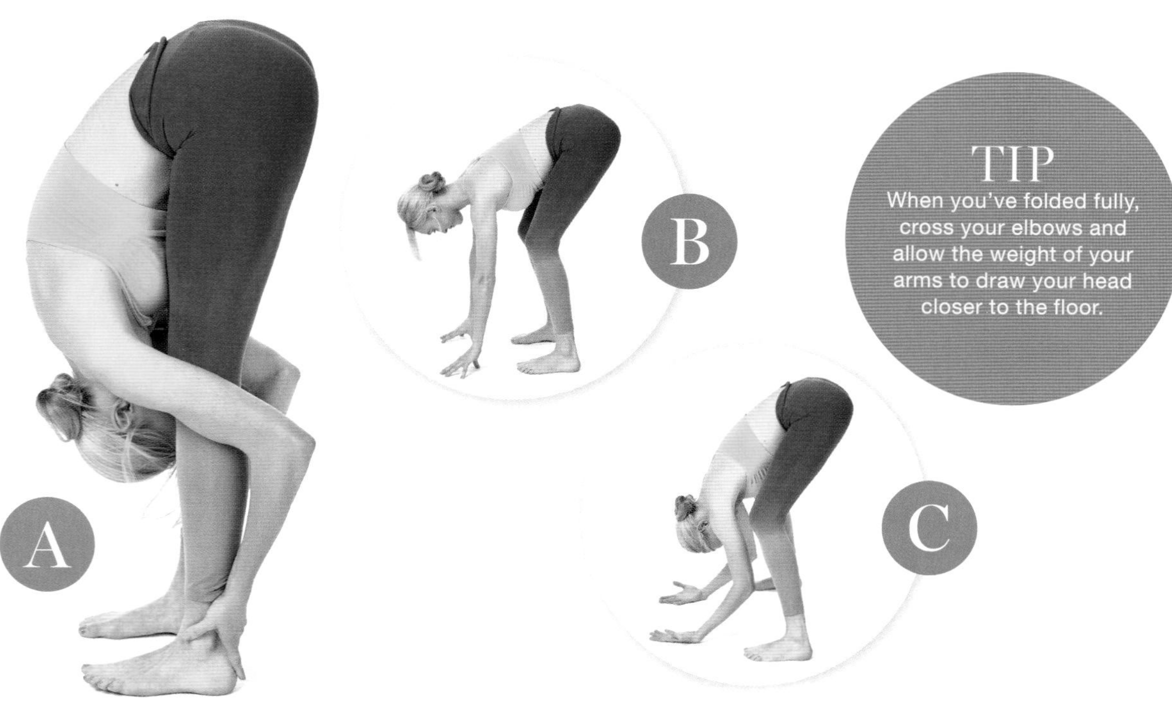

TIP

When you've folded fully, cross your elbows and allow the weight of your arms to draw your head closer to the floor.

SUPPORTED HEADSTAND

SALAMBA SIRSASANA

- Come onto all-fours, interlace your fingers and rest your forearms on the floor, elbows beneath your shoulders.
- Place your crown on the floor, with the back of your head resting against your cupped hands. Draw your elbows towards each other and take your shoulders down your spine to maintain space around your neck.
- Straighten your legs, come up onto tip toes and raise your tailbone towards the ceiling. Walk you toes as far forwards as you can, drawing your abdominals to your spine as you do so. Allow your forearms, rather than your head, to take most of your weight (A).
- Breathing evenly, continue walking forwards until your hips are stacked over your shoulders, then bend your knees and lift your legs, taking your knees towards your chest (B). Once you're confident of your balance, straighten your legs (C).
- Stay in the pose for up to five minutes, then exhale, and slowly release your legs to the floor.
- Rest for a few minutes in Child's pose (p34).

GOOD FOR

- Calms your mind
- Builds concentration
- Boosts energy
- Strengthens your core, arms and shoulders

TIP

Engage your core to help you maintain your balance. Start by practising against a wall, gradually moving further away as your skill and confidence grows.

A

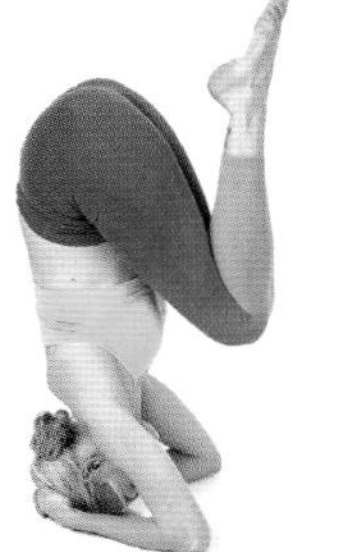

B

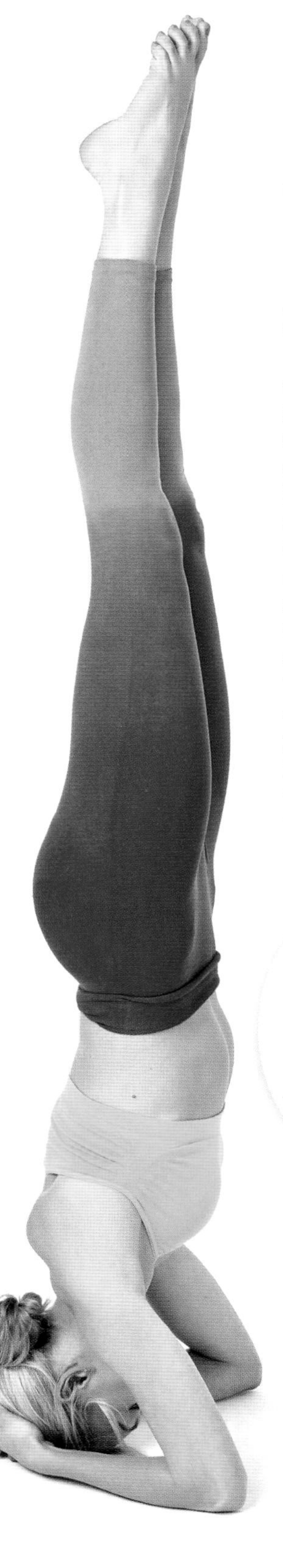

C

TREE POSE
VRKSASANA

● From Mountain pose (p44), transfer your weight onto your left leg. Spread your toes and ground through the base of your big and little toes.
● Maintain a micro-bend in your left knee and place the sole of your right foot against the inner seam of your left calf or thigh (but not on the knee). Rest your hands on your hips while you establish your balance, focusing on a point straight ahead of you.
● Draw your right knee out to the side, your tailbone towards the floor and your belly to your spine. Root down as you lift out of your waist and up through your crown. Bring your hands to prayer position at your heart (A) then, if you feel well balanced, slowly glide your hands overhead (B).
● Take five deep breaths, then exhale and gently lower your hands and foot and repeat on the other side.
● Beginners, place your foot low to begin with (C).

GOOD FOR

● Mental and physical balance
● Stretches your groin, chest and shoulders
● Calms your mind
● Grounding

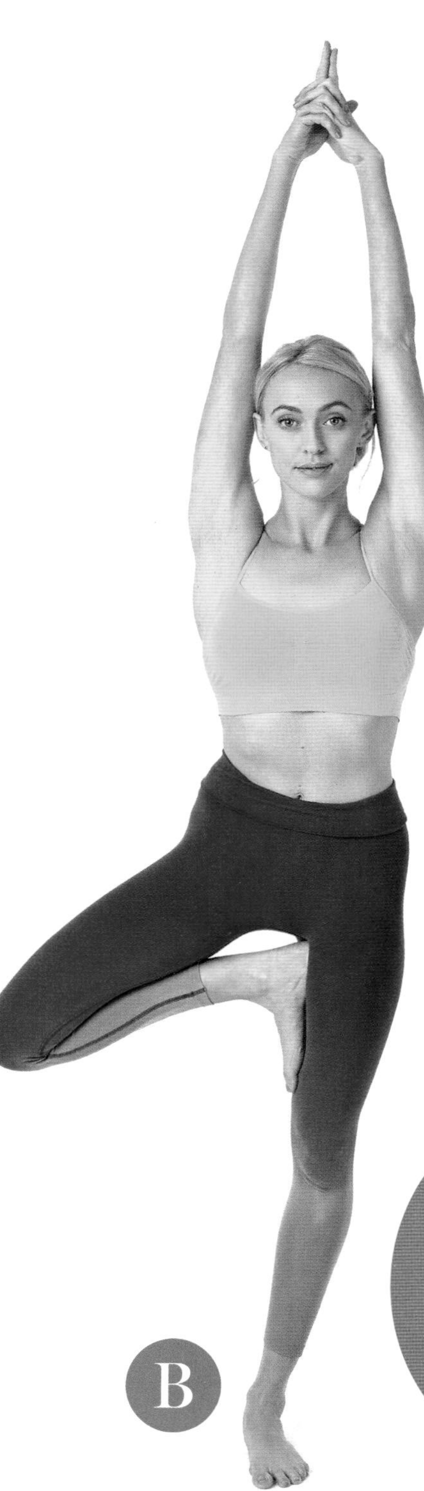

C

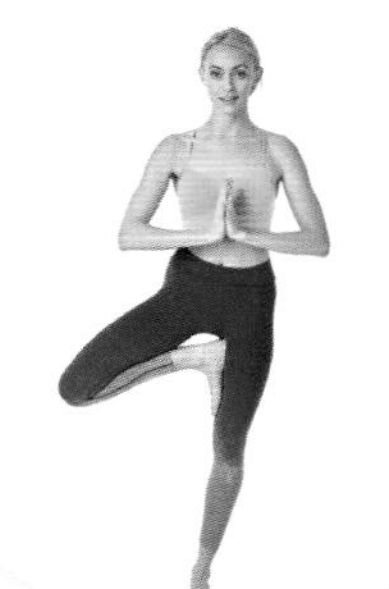

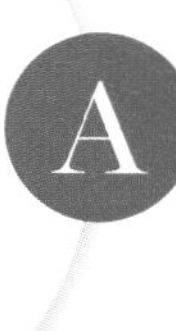

TIP

If your foot slips down your thigh, focus on pressing the sole of your foot into your thigh at the same time as pressing your thigh against the sole of your foot. This will help to stabilise you.

TRIANGLE POSE
UTTHITA TRIKONASANA

● Stand sideways on the centre of your mat and take a moment to arrive in your body, breathing deeply into your belly. When you feel ready, step your feet a leg's length apart.
● Turn your right foot out 90 degrees and your left foot in 15 degrees. Align your heels (or right heel to left instep), then root down through your big and little toes, the centre of your heels and the outer edge of your left foot. Breathe.
● Place your hands on your hips and tilt your right hip down and your left hip back and up. On an inhale, extend your arms out to shoulder height. As you exhale, keep your arms parallel to the floor as you reach your right hand outwards as far as is comfortable, before releasing it down to rest where it naturally lands, on your calf or ankle.
● On your next inhale, float your left arm overhead and rotate open your chest, so your left shoulder is above the right and your arms are in a straight line. Let your gaze rest on the floor, directly ahead or, if comfortable for your neck, turn your head to look up at your top hand.
● Breathe into the pose, making micro-adjustments, until you feel rooted but open, using your in-breath to ground through your feet and lengthen your side body, and your out-breath to release further into the twist. Rest in your final position for five to 10 breaths, breathing deeply into your belly.
● When you're ready, root through your feet and inhale up to standing, then exhale as you lower your arms and step your feet together. Pause for a moment to register the effects of the pose, then repeat on the other side.

GOOD FOR
● Relieves stiffness in your legs, hips and neck
● Relieves tension in your back
● Opens your side body/improves your breathing
● Eases menstrual symptoms

WARRIOR II
VIRABHADRASANA II

● After taking a few breaths to still your mind and become present to this moment, step your feet wide, turning your right foot out 90 degrees and your left foot in 15 degrees. Align your right heel with your left heel or, for beginners, your left instep. Spread your toes and root through your big and little toes and the outside edge of your left foot.

● With your weight balanced evenly between both feet, your pelvis in neutral and facing the long side of your mat, inhale to raise your arms to the sides, palms facing the floor. Lengthen from your centre to beyond your fingertips.

● On an exhale, bend your right leg to take your knee directly over your ankle, keeping a micro-bend in your left leg.

● Breathing evenly, draw your navel to your spine, open your chest and slide your shoulders down your spine. If comfortable, turn your head to gaze along your front arm, beyond your middle finger (A).

● Take five breaths into your belly, draw your inner thighs together and feel how the strength of your lower body brings a freedom to your upper body. When you feel ready, exhale, gently lower your hands and step your feet together.

● Pause for a moment to register the effects of the pose before repeating on the other side.

GOOD FOR

● Increases focus and determination
● Strengthens your legs
● Grounding
● Helps you connect to your strength

VARIATION
REVERSE WARRIOR (B)

● From Warrior II, inhale as you slide your back arm down your back thigh, and raise your front arm overhead, gently arching your spine laterally. Root your feet down and lift your torso up on each inhale, feeling your side body open and, as you exhale, arc a little further into the backbend. Take five breaths, then change sides.

TIP
Your spine is vertical in this pose. If you find yourself leaning forwards, extend your back hand towards the back of the mat.
A
B

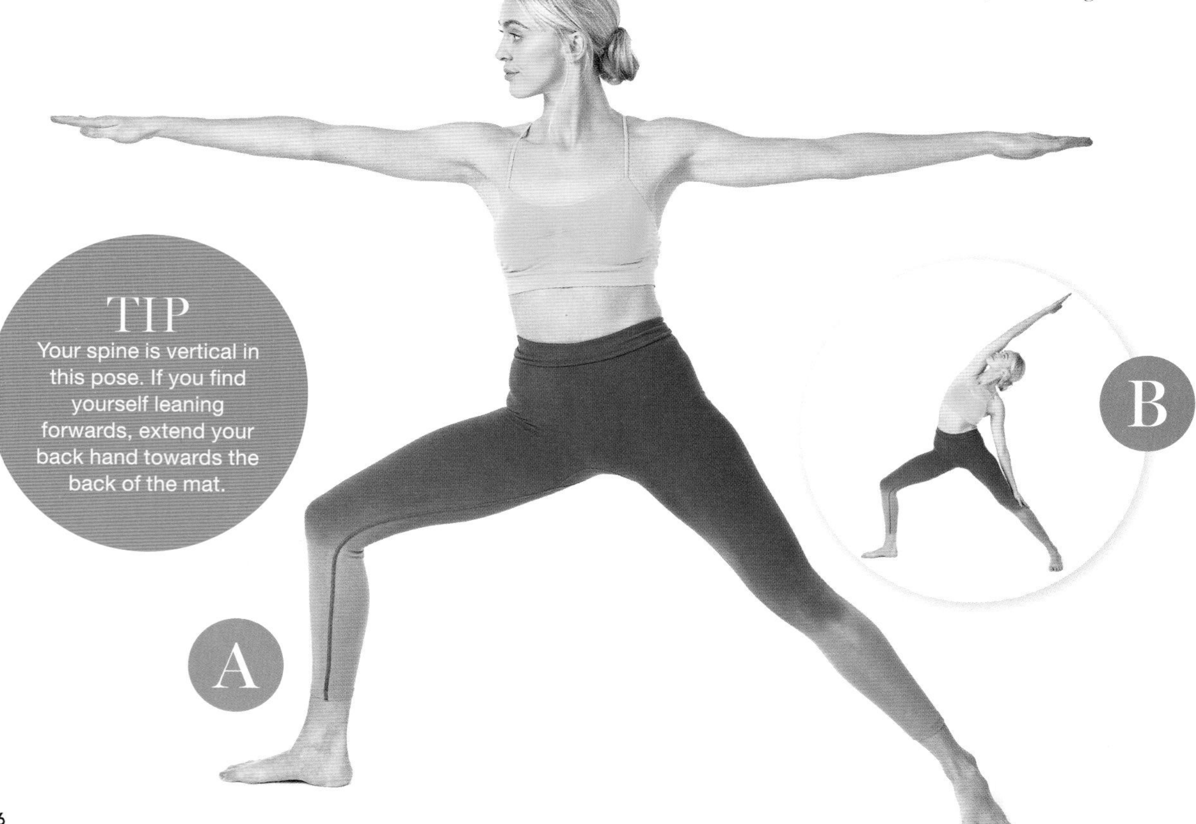

WARRIOR III
VIRABHADRASANA III

- From Mountain pose (p44) inhale, transfer your weight to your right foot and raise your arms overhead.
- On an exhale, raise your left leg backwards as you draw your navel to your spine and tilt your body forwards, leading with your chest.
- Engage the thigh muscles of your right leg and rotate the outside edge of your left thigh down to keep your hips level and flex your left ankle.
- Continue tilting forwards until your legs, torso and arms are parallel to the floor, reaching from your centre right through to your toes and fingertips.
- Take five to 10 breaths, then repeat on the other side.

GOOD FOR
- Balance
- Strengthening your ankles and legs
- Focus
- Core strength

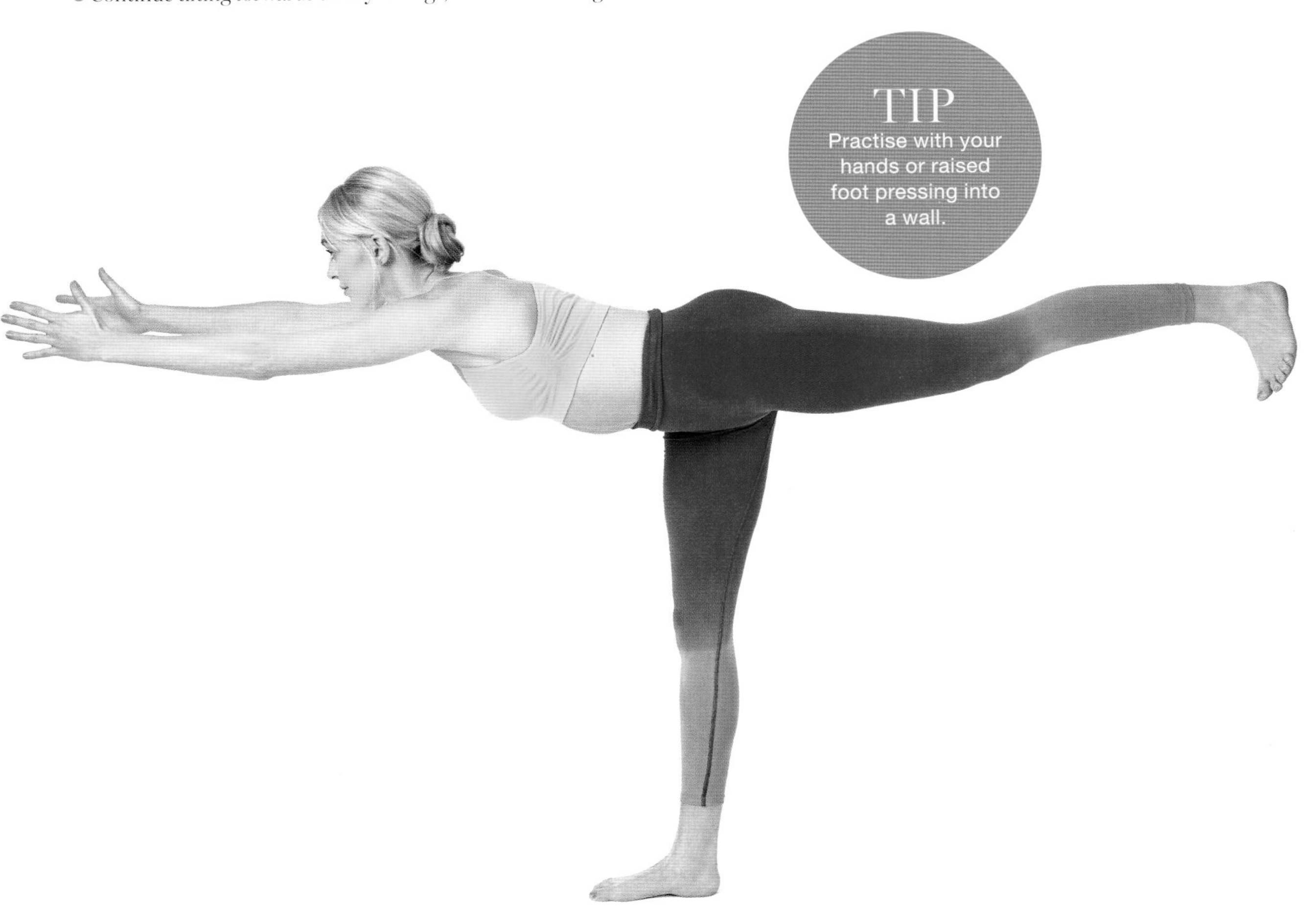

TIP
Practise with your hands or raised foot pressing into a wall.

WHEEL POSE
URDHVA DHANURASANA

- Lie on your back, knees bent and heels close to your buttocks. Place your palms on the floor beside your shoulders, fingertips pointing to your feet, elbows in and pointing upwards (A).
- On an inhale, press your hands and feet into the floor and raise your hips up and back. Raise your head and rest your crown on the floor. Check your elbows are shoulder-width-apart (B). Exhale.
- On your next inhale, press into the floor and straighten your arms and legs to lift your body.
- Release your neck and imagine your body being lifted up by the navel (C). Take five deep breaths, then lower on an exhale by gently bending your arms and legs.

A

B

GOOD FOR

- Boosts energy
- Soothes stress
- Strengthens your thighs, shoulders, arms, wrists and spine

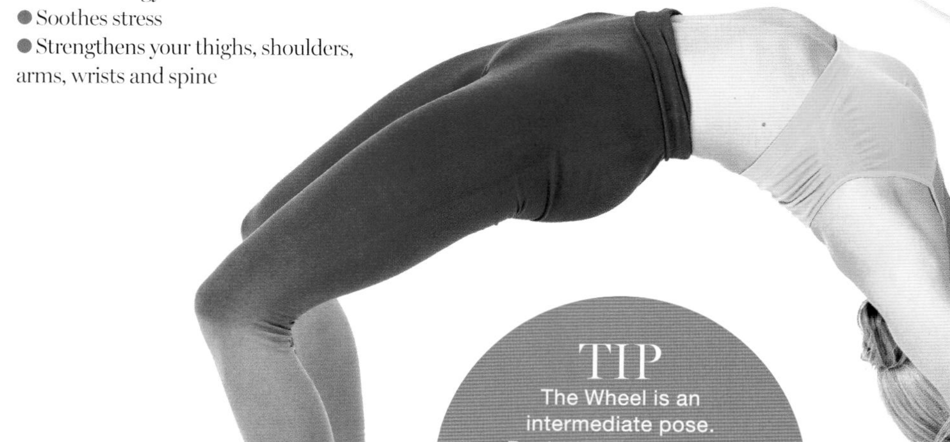

TIP

The Wheel is an intermediate pose. Beginners, practise by placing two blocks against a wall and alternate resting your hands or your feet on them, to lessen the depth of the backbend.

WIDE-LEGGED STANDING FORWARD FOLD

PRASARITA PADOTTANASANA

- Standing sideways on your mat, step your feet wide, inner edges parallel. Spread your toes, lift your inner arches and root through the outer edges of your feet.
- With your hands on your hips, inhale and lengthen your spine out of your waist. On an exhale, fold forwards from your hips with a flat back. When your spine is parallel to the floor, place your hands on the mat, shoulder-width apart, fingers forwards.
- On each inhale, lengthen your spine, on each exhale fold a little deeper, lowering the crown of your head to the floor. As your head gets close to the mat, move your hands between your feet, fingers spread wide and forearms vertical. Soften your neck.
- Draw up your kneecaps and engage your thighs, keep releasing your upper body downwards and ground through your hands to draw your shoulders away from your neck (A). Breathe deeply and evenly for up to 10 breaths.
- To return to standing, place your hands on your hips and inhale as you slowly return to vertical.

VARIATION 1 (B) & (C)

- For an intense side stretch, walk your hands over to your right foot, opening the left side of your spine. Take five deep breaths, then walk your hands over to your left foot.

VARIATION 2 (D)

- Walk your hands forwards, shoulder-width apart and fingers spread. Root through the base of your fingers and draw your arms into your arm sockets and your shoulders down your spine. Keep your neck in line with your spine, and breathe deeply for five to 10 breaths.

GOOD FOR

- Calms your mind
- Removes fatigue
- Relieves backache
- Stretches your legs and spine

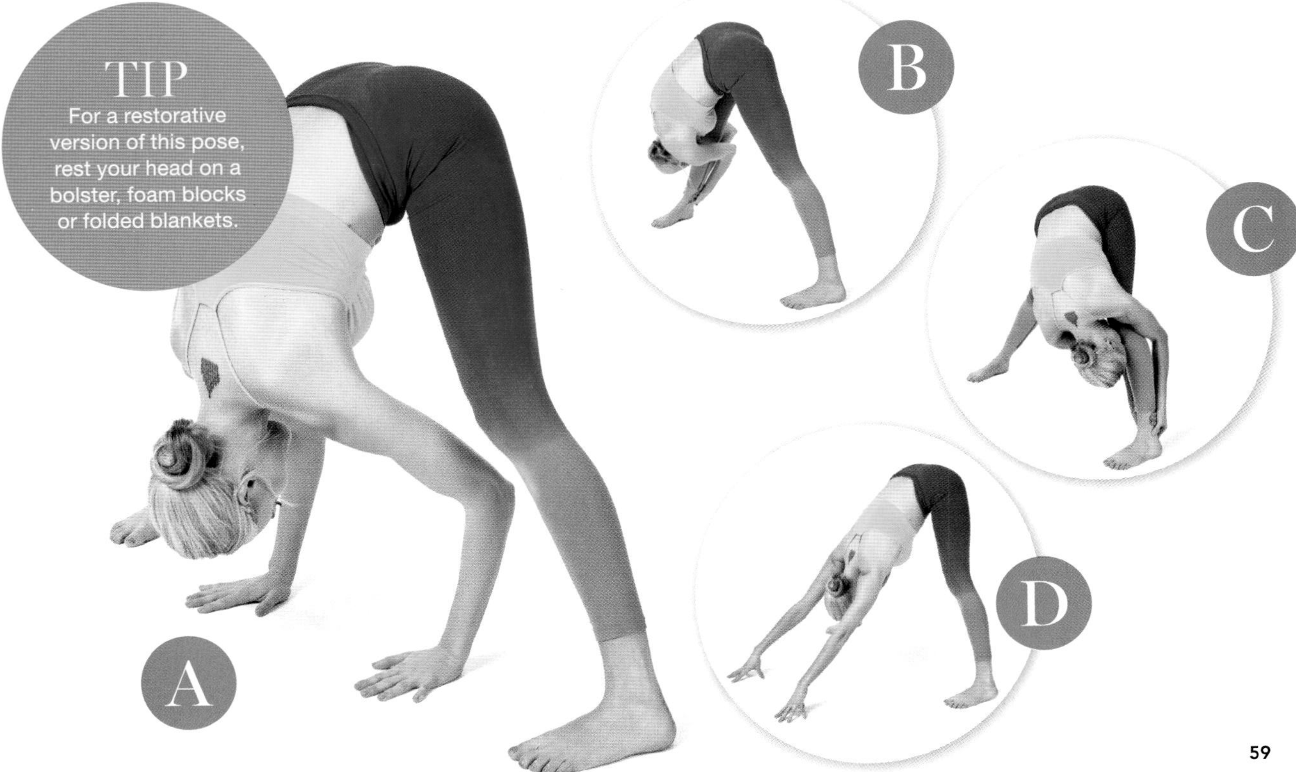

TIP

For a restorative version of this pose, rest your head on a bolster, foam blocks or folded blankets.

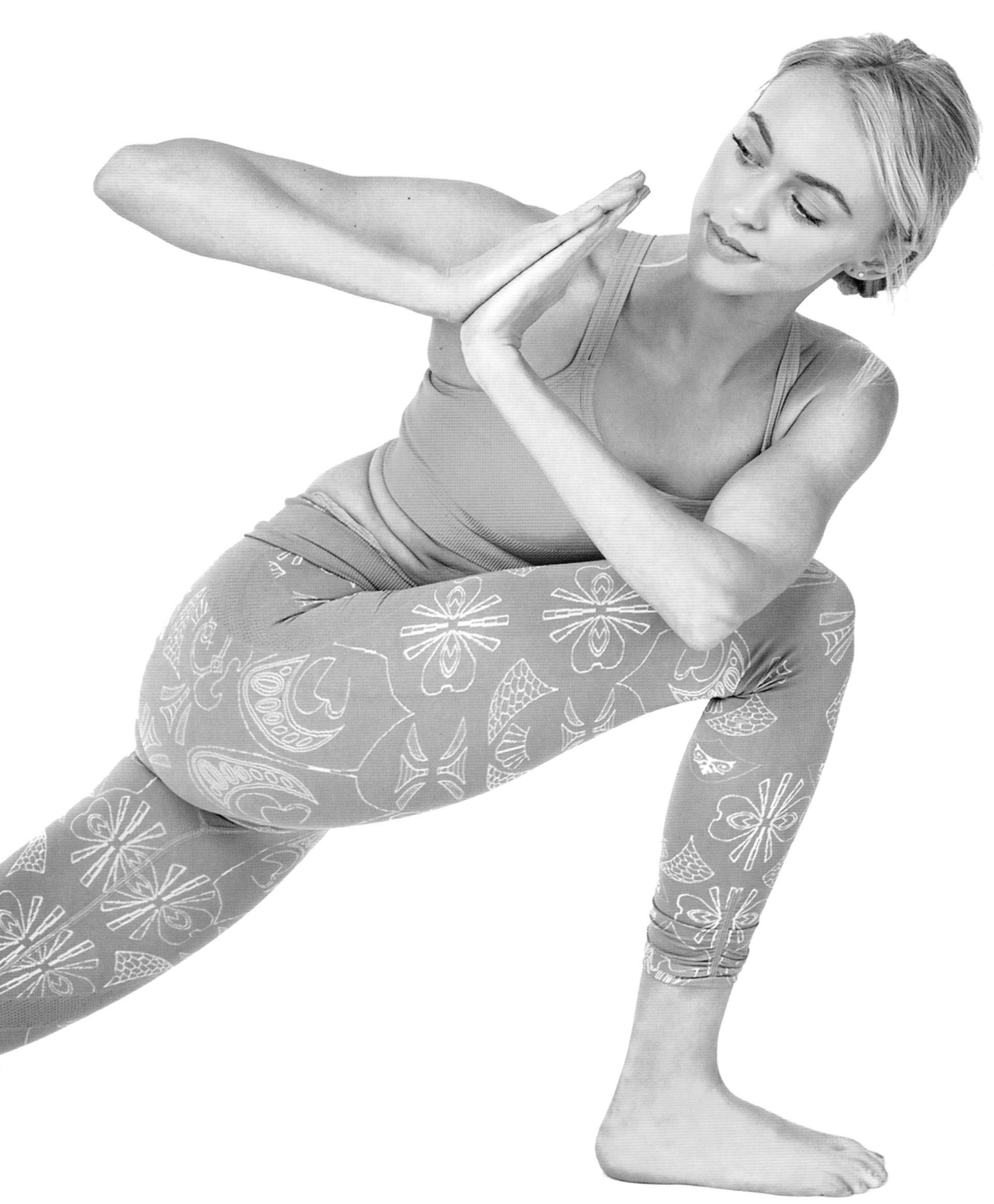

PM POSES

Now that you've learned the foundation poses, it's time to enjoy the benefits of the evening postures. Based on yin and restorative yoga, these calming poses will stretch your connective tissue, soothe your mind and bring you into a deeply relaxed state. Move as far as is comfortable into the stretches until you meet your 'edge' then wait for your muscles to gradually soften before releasing deeper into the pose. Enjoy!

BUTTERFLY

- Sit on your mat, checking that your weight is evenly distributed between your sitting bones. Bend your knees and bring the soles of your feet together, then let them fall out to the side like a butterfly. After a moment or two, slide your feet forwards to make a diamond shape with your legs.
- Grasp your feet with your hands and fold forwards letting your weight come onto the front of your sitting bones as you allow your spine to gently drape forwards. Let your neck release and your forehead drop towards your hands. Rest for a while here, then as you feel your muscles soften and release, sink a little deeper into the pose.
- Spend three to five minutes here, then inhale and engage your abdomen to come back up to sitting. Slowly stretch your legs in front of you and lean back on your hands, gently arching your back as a counterpose to the forward bend.

GOOD FOR

- Regulates periods
- Releases tension in your spine
- Opens your hips
- Calms your brain

TIP

Place a block under each knee to minimise stress on your groin. You can also rest your head on a bolster for an even more restorative pose.

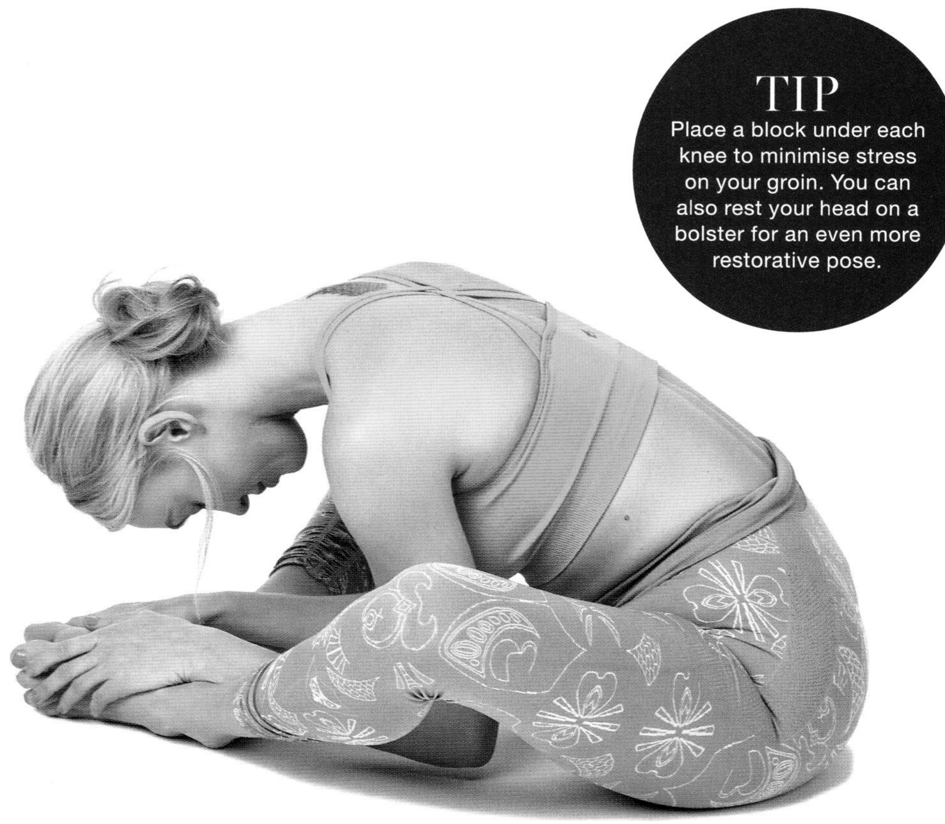

CAT PULLING ITS TAIL

● Sit with your legs straight in front of you and twist to your left to rest on your left elbow, hand supporting your head. Keeping your left leg straight for a moment, reach your right leg forwards and bend your knee to 90 degrees so your knee is in line with your hip.

● Bend your left leg and grasp hold of your toes with your right hand. Pull your hand towards you at the same times as pulling your foot away from your hand. This will create a deep stretch in your left quadriceps.

● Rest here for three to five minutes, then release your bottom foot and roll onto your stomach. Pause for a moment before repeating on the other side.

GOOD FOR

- Deeply relaxing
- Aids insomnia
- Stretches your quads
- Eases tension in your lower back

VARIATION (B)

● For a deep reclining twist, from Cat pulling its tail, release your right shoulder down to the floor, bring your left arm into cactus arms, and straighten your top leg. Enjoy the sensation of the stretch for up to five minutes, then repeat on the other side.

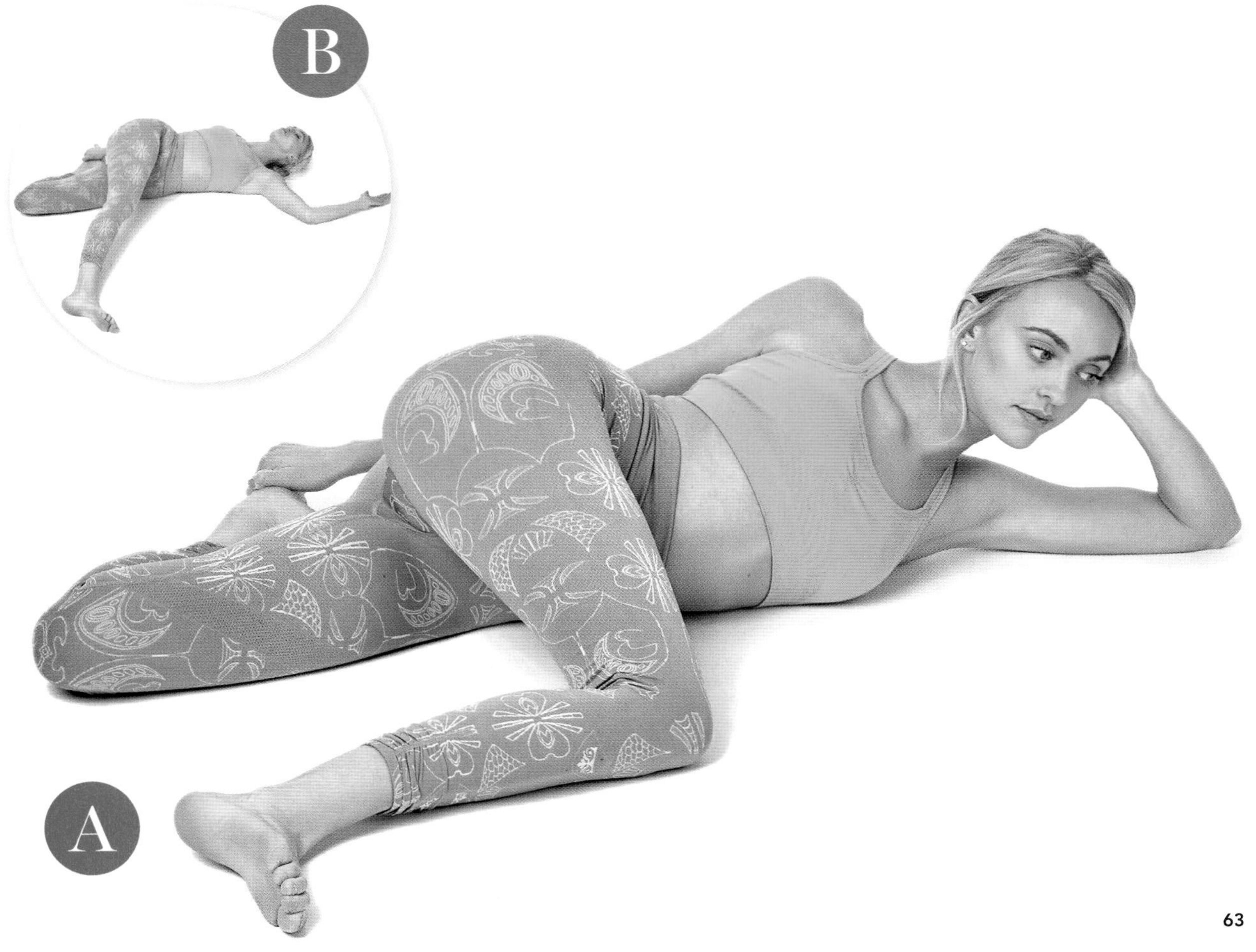

HAPPY BABY

- Lie on your back and take a moment to centre yourself. Take three deep breaths, releasing any tension on the exhale.
- When you feel ready, bend your knees deeply, take hold of your outer feet with each hand and open your knees, allowing them to release down towards your armpits.
- Flex your ankles, with your soles facing the ceiling, and bring your calves to vertical. Feel the stretch and deep release in your lower back.
- Tuck in your chin to lengthen your neck, and draw your shoulders down your spine to create space around your neck. Reach your tailbone forwards to lengthen your spine.
- Stay here for 10-20 deep slow breaths, then rock gently from side to side before releasing your feet to the floor.

GOOD FOR

- Relieves stress
- Opens your inner and outer thighs
- Eases lower back tension
- Uplifting

TIP

If you can't reach your feet comfortably, wrap a strap around the balls of your feet and hold one end in each hand. As your flexibility increases you can 'walk' your hands up the strap until you eventually don't need it.

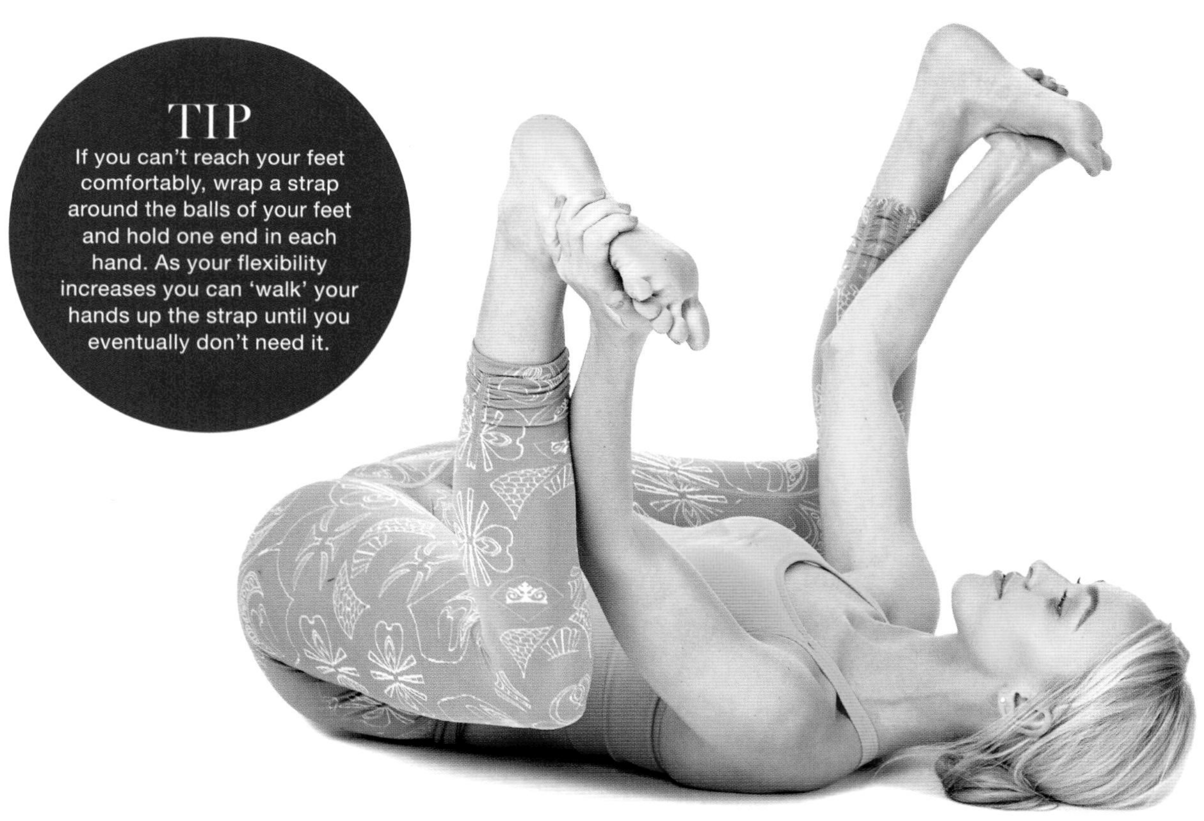

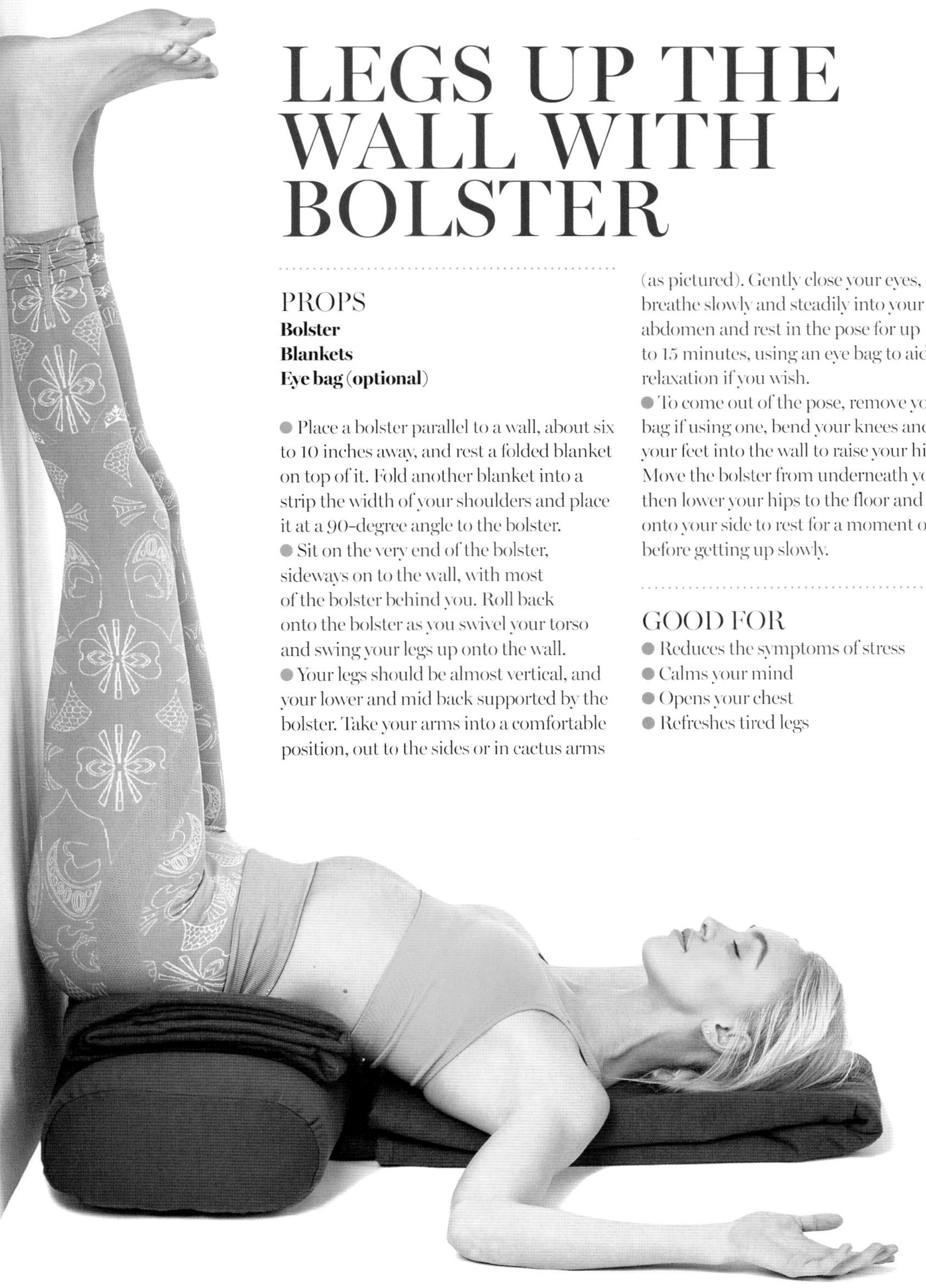

LEGS UP THE WALL WITH BOLSTER

PROPS

Bolster
Blankets
Eye bag (optional)

- Place a bolster parallel to a wall, about six to 10 inches away, and rest a folded blanket on top of it. Fold another blanket into a strip the width of your shoulders and place it at a 90-degree angle to the bolster.
- Sit on the very end of the bolster, sideways on to the wall, with most of the bolster behind you. Roll back onto the bolster as you swivel your torso and swing your legs up onto the wall.
- Your legs should be almost vertical, and your lower and mid back supported by the bolster. Take your arms into a comfortable position, out to the sides or in cactus arms (as pictured). Gently close your eyes, breathe slowly and steadily into your abdomen and rest in the pose for up to 15 minutes, using an eye bag to aid relaxation if you wish.
- To come out of the pose, remove your eye bag if using one, bend your knees and press your feet into the wall to raise your hips. Move the bolster from underneath you, then lower your hips to the floor and roll onto your side to rest for a moment or two before getting up slowly.

GOOD FOR

- Reduces the symptoms of stress
- Calms your mind
- Opens your chest
- Refreshes tired legs

MOUNTAIN BROOK

PROPS:

Bolster
Blankets
Eye bag (optional)

- Fold two blankets into strips and another into a rectangle, rolling up one edge to make a support for your neck. Arrange the props on your mat as in the image, then lie on your back, with the blankets and bolster supporting you.
- Make any adjustments you need, decreasing or increasing the height of the blankets, to ensure that your neck is fully supported, your head tilting gently back and your chest open, but not strained.
- Extend your arms to the sides, palms facing upwards and gently close your eyes, using an eye bag if you wish.
- Breathing normally, scan your body and allow any tension to melt away on the out breath. Notice your jaw, temples and shoulders, your belly, hips and legs, letting your body feel heavier and heavier as it sinks into the mat.
- Rest here for up to five minutes, then remove your eye bag, softly stretch your whole body and gently roll onto your side before coming up to sitting.

GOOD FOR

- Aids breathing
- Opens your shoulders after sitting at a desk
- Reduces fatigue
- Lifts your mood

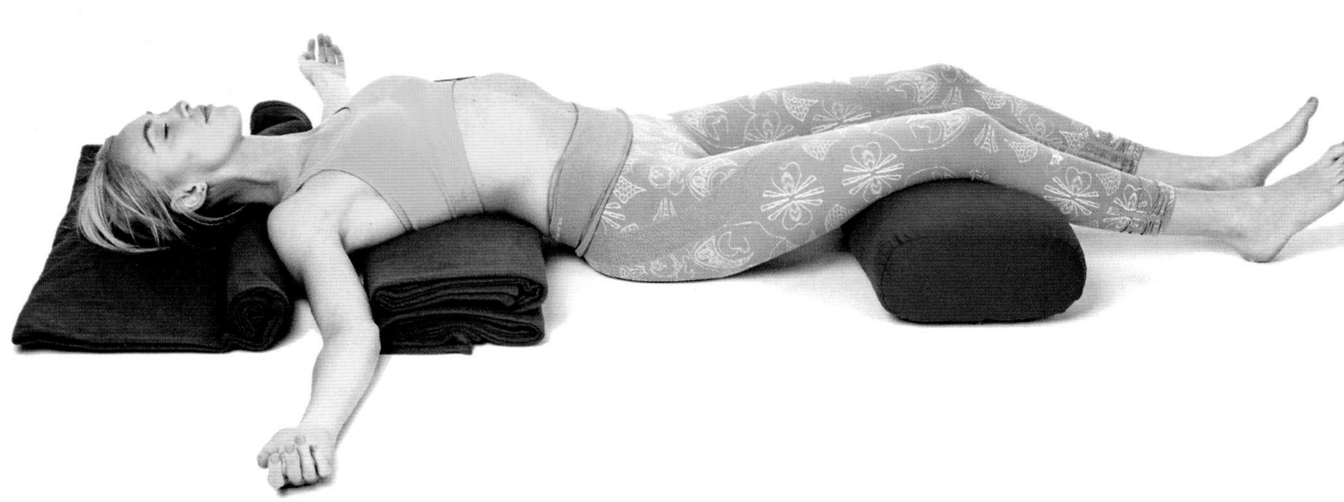

RELAXATION POSE

PROPS

Bolster
Blanket
Eye bag (optional)

● Place a bolster crosswise about a quarter of the way down your mat and roll one side of a folded blanket at the other end. Have another blanket and an eye bag close by.

● Rather than lean back to lie down, which places a strain on your abdomen, from kneeling, lower down onto your right buttock and place your right hand out to the side. Use your hands and forearms to help you lower down onto your right side, then roll over onto your back.

● Take your arms to your sides, palms facing up, and bring your chin slightly lower than your forehead, to quieten the frontal lobes of your brain.

● Cover your eyes with an eye bag and your body with a blanket.

● Breathing softly and deeply into your belly, scan your body from head to toe, consciously letting go of any tension on an out-breath. Relax your temples and release your lower jaw. Lengthen the back of your neck and let go of any tension around your lips. Let your eyeballs sink into your eye sockets, and your eyelids be heavy.

● Continue travelling down your body, letting your muscles melt into your bones and your bones sink into the mat. Let your thoughts recede and your mind become still, resting here for up to 20 minutes.

● When ready to come out of the pose, take your attention to your breath, then gently bring some movement back to your body. Wriggle your fingers and toes, take your arms overhead and stretch from your hands to your feet. Bring the soles of your feet onto the bolster, take your hips to the left and roll over to your right hand side. Rest in a foetal position for a few breaths, then press your left hand into the floor to help you come up to a sitting position.

GOOD FOR

● Lowers blood pressure and heart rate
● Reduces fatigue
● Improves sleep
● Releases muscular tension

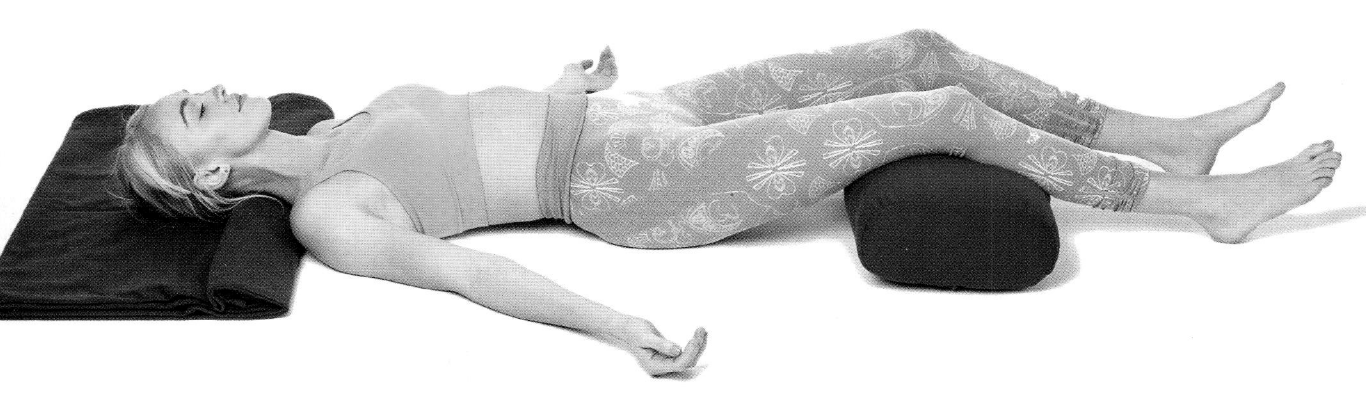

RESTORATIVE BUTTERFLY

PROPS

Two bolsters
Four folded blankets
Strap
Eye bag (optional)

● Place the bolsters and blankets on your mat as pictured, and have a yoga strap nearby.

● Sit cross-legged, with your buttocks against the short edge of the lengthwise bolster. Place the centre of an open strap around your lower back, bring the ends forwards and let them fall over your thighs and calves. Take one end and loop it under the outside edges of both feet and adjust the strap so the buckle won't press against your legs when you lie down.

● Bring the soles of your feet together and let your knees fall out to the sides, then tighten the strap as needed.

● Rest one hand on either side of your buttocks, inhale, then as you exhale, slowly lower your spine onto the lengthwise bolster, resting your head on a block or folded blanket if needed so your neck is comfortable. Place your arms out to the sides, palms up.

● Make any minor adjustments you need, so there is no strain on any part of your body, perhaps adding a thin block or folded blanket beneath your buttocks to lessen the curve of your lower back.

● Gently close your eyes, connect to your breath and surrender your weight to the earth. Rest here for as long as is comfortable for you, up to 10 minutes. Then gently bring your knees together, shift your bottom to the left, let your knees fall to your right and slowly roll your body over to the right, so your back comes off the bolster. Pause here for a moment, before using your hands to gently bring you up to sitting.

GOOD FOR

● Calms your nervous system
● Regulates your blood pressure
● Opens your hips and heart area
● Works on your liver, kidney and spleen meridians

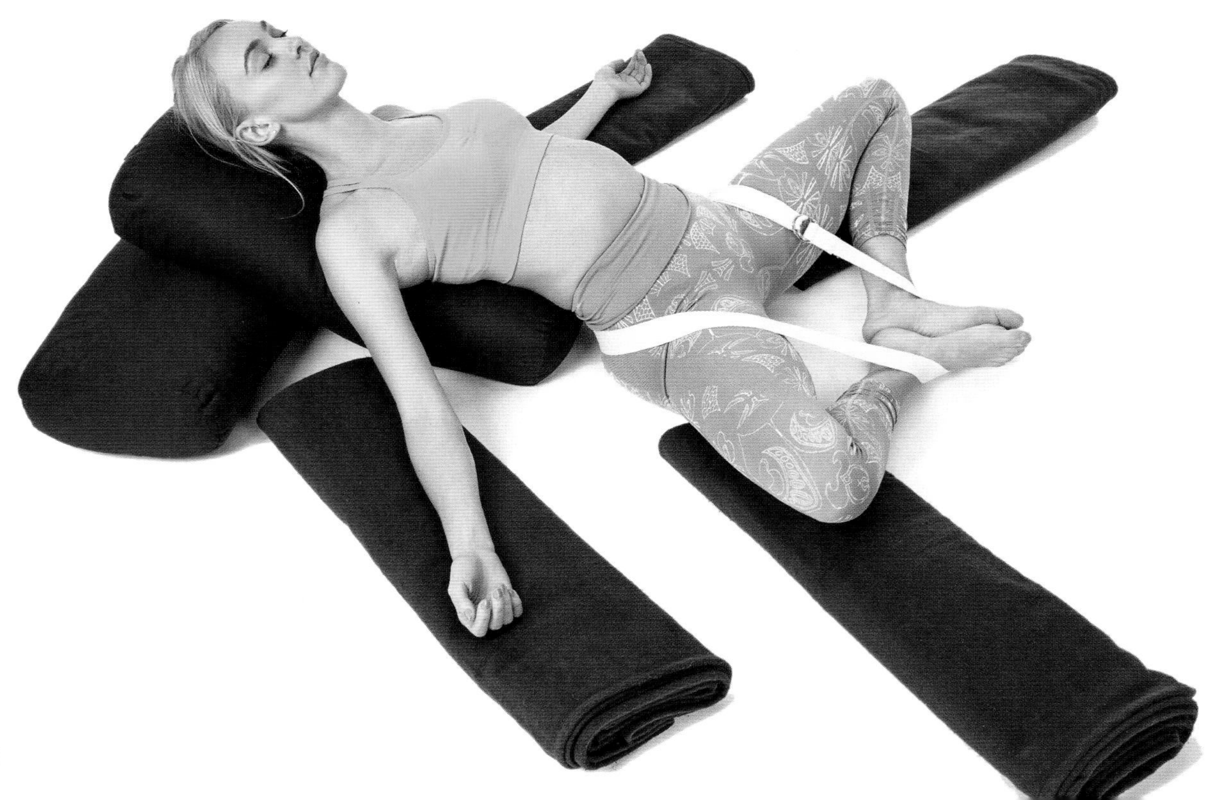

RESTORATIVE CHILD'S POSE

PROPS

Bolster
Blankets
Sandbag (optional)

● Cover your mat with a blanket for extra padding, then kneel down with the bolster lengthwise between your thighs and your ankles pointing directly backwards. Sit back on your heels and notice how your knees or ankles feel. If you feel any discomfort, try the suggestions in the tip below.

● Take a couple of slow, gentle breaths, then gently fold forwards to rest your chest over the bolster. Allow your tailbone to release towards your heels to lengthen your lower back. You can place a sandbag over your sacrum to help your muscles relax more deeply.

● Rest your head to one side, raising it on a folded blanket if this feels more comfortable for your neck, then gently draw your chin in towards your chest, making sure you can breathe easily. Extend your arms forwards, wrap your arms around the bolster or take your hands back towards your hips, whichever feels right for your body in this moment. Draw your shoulders away from your ears to create space around your neck.

● Allow your breathing to settle. Let your jaw relax and your belly soften. Allow any tension to melt away as you surrender your weight into the bolster. Rest here for up to three minutes, turning your head to face the opposite direction half-way through.

● To come out of the pose, place your hands under your shoulders and inhale as you gently press your hands into the mat to help raise your torso. Move the bolster to one side and rest in a comfortable seated position for a few breaths.

GOOD FOR

● Calms your nervous system
● Soothes your mind
● Deeply relaxing
● Aids insomnia

TIP

If your knees or ankles feel uncomfortable, try placing a folded towel onto the back of your knees and a rolled towel under the front of your ankles.

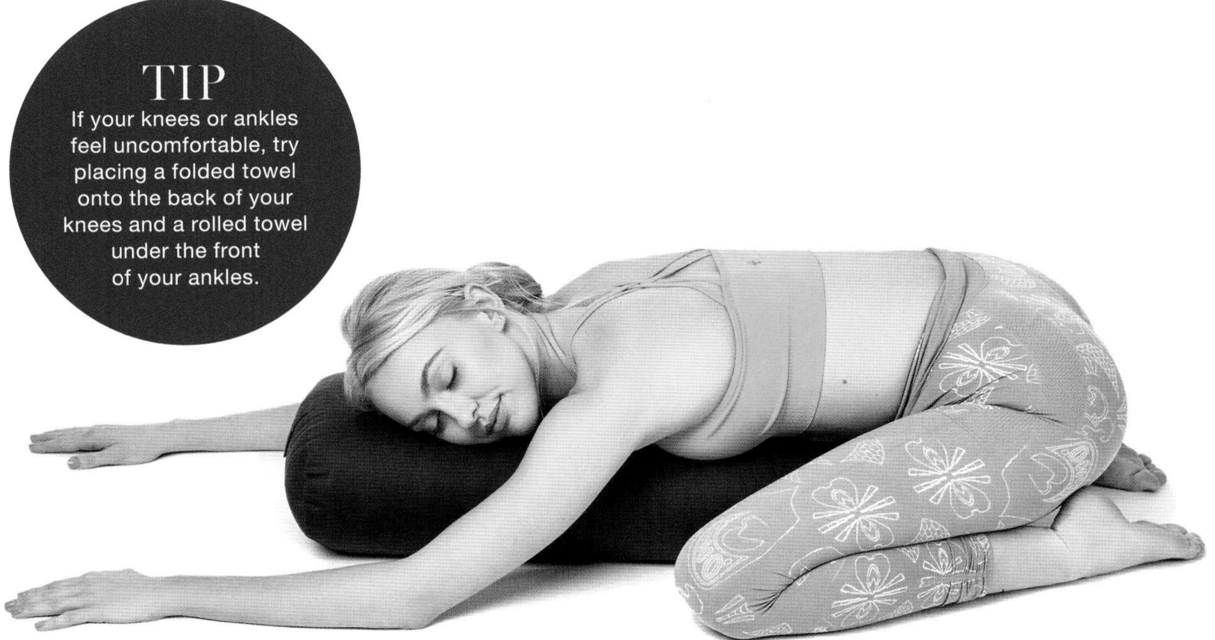

RESTORATIVE TWIST

PROPS

Bolster
Blankets

- Cover your mat with a blanket, place a bolster lengthwise down the centre and have another folded blanket close by. Snuggle your left buttock into the short end of the bolster, so your left thigh is parallel to it, your knees are bent and feet resting to your left.
- Take a couple of slow, gentle breaths, then inhale to lengthen your spine and, as you exhale, twist to your left and walk your hands forwards as you gently fold from your hips to rest the centre of your chest over the bolster.
- Turn your head to face your left and rest your left cheek on the bolster, raising it on a folded blanket if this feels more comfortable for your neck.
- Draw your shoulder blades down your back to create space around your neck. Relax your arms comfortably on the floor, elbows bent and palms facing down.
- Breathe softly and evenly into your back and side ribs, releasing deeper into the twist on the exhale, as you surrender to gravity and allow yourself to be fully supported by the bolster.
- After one to two minutes, change sides. Place your hands under your shoulders and inhale as you gently press your hands into the mat to help raise your torso. Swap your knees to the opposite side, so your outer right thigh rests against the bolster, and lower down, this time twisting to your right.
- When you're ready to come out, root through your hands to lift up, then move the bolster to one side and rest in a comfortable seated position for a few breaths.

GOOD FOR

- Relieves tension in your upper back
- Expands your intercostal muscles to aid breathing
- Calms your mind

TIP

To avoid straining your back when you come out of the pose, turn your head to face your knees for one or two breaths, then come up slowly.

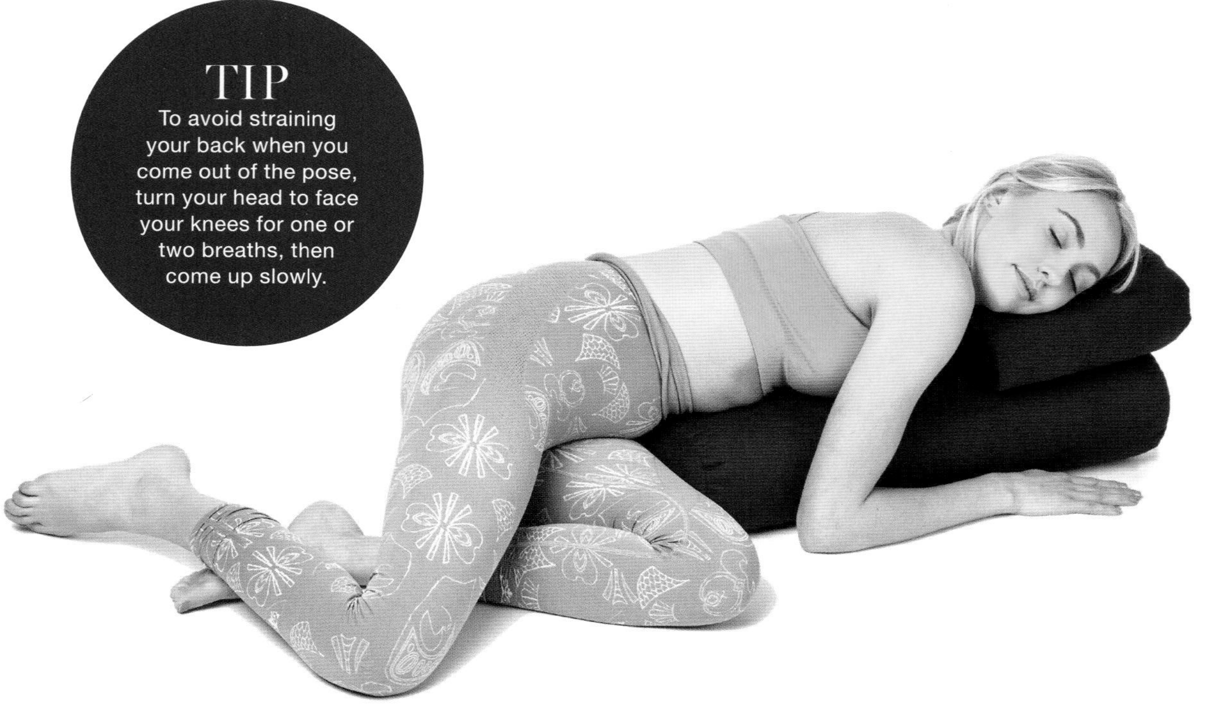

SADDLE

- Kneel up on your mat with your knees slightly apart, tops of your feet flat on the floor, and gently ease your buttocks between your feet.
- Take your hands behind you and rest your fingertips on the floor, leaning backwards as you do. Arch your upper back, and tilt your tailbone back towards your lumbar spine, to deeply arch your back.
- If it's not too much of a strain on your quadriceps (front thighs), gently lower onto your forearms. Allow your knees to remain apart, to avoid stressing the joints (A), and rest in the pose for three to five minutes. If comfortable, you can lie back on your mat or on a bolster.
- To come out of the posture, gently engage your abdominals and come back to keeling. Rest for a moment or two with your eyes closed before coming back up to standing.

VARIATION (B)

- If Saddle is too demanding on your knees, try keeping one leg straight and the other bent, switching sides after a few minutes. As you gradually increase the flexibility of your quads you'll be able to work with both knees bent.

GOOD FOR

- Opens your hip flexors
- Stretches your quads

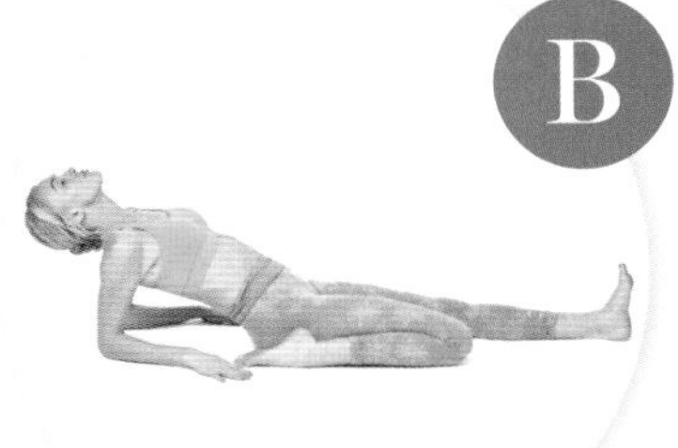

TIP

If you have tight ankles, place a cushion under them, and if your knees are uncomfortable, place a rolled blanket behind your bent knee.

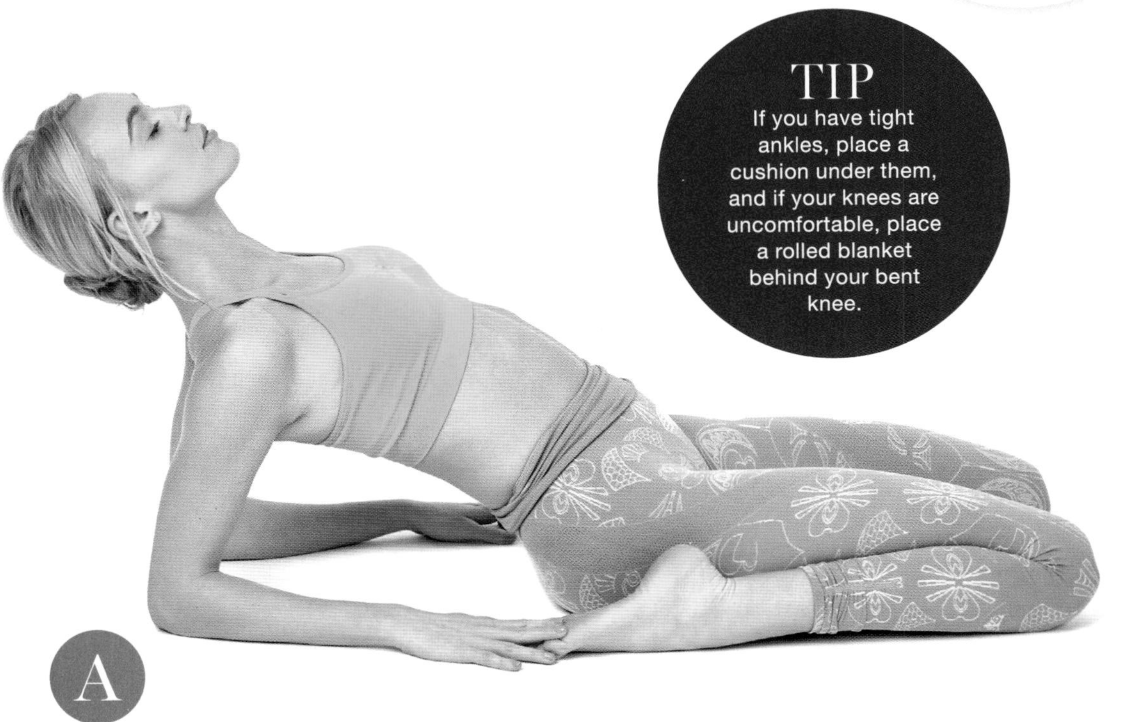

SHOELACE

● Spend a moment or two in Child's pose (p69) to let your breath settle, then when you feel ready, come up onto all-fours. Lift your left knee, take it back slightly and cross it over your right calf to place it outside your right shin. Spread your feet away from each other, then exhale as you gently lower your bottom to sit between your feet.

● Root evenly through both sitting bones. If one side doesn't touch the floor, place a folded blanket or thin block beneath it. Holding a foot in each hand, guide your feet as far back as is comfortable, keeping one knee above the other. If your bottom leg is uncomfortable keep it extended in front of you.

● Take a couple of breaths to acclimatise to the stretch; root through your sitting bones as you open your chest, lengthen the back of your neck and lift through your crown on the in-breath, allowing your weight to sink down on the out-breath.

● Softly inhale as you float your arms out to the sides, shoulder height. Exhale and cross your arms in front of you, your left elbow on top of your right, then intertwine your forearms to bring your palms together, fingertips pointing up and thumbs facing you. Gently close your eyes.

● Take a few gentle Ocean breaths (p98), expanding into your back and side body, then let your breath find its natural rhythm. Settle into a sense of stillness, resting in the pose for up to two minutes.

● Gently release your arms, and, with great care, your legs, then pause for a moment in a comfortable seated position before repeating on the other side.

GOOD FOR

- Deeply stills your mind
- Calms anxiety
- Removes tension from your shoulders
- Strong hip opener

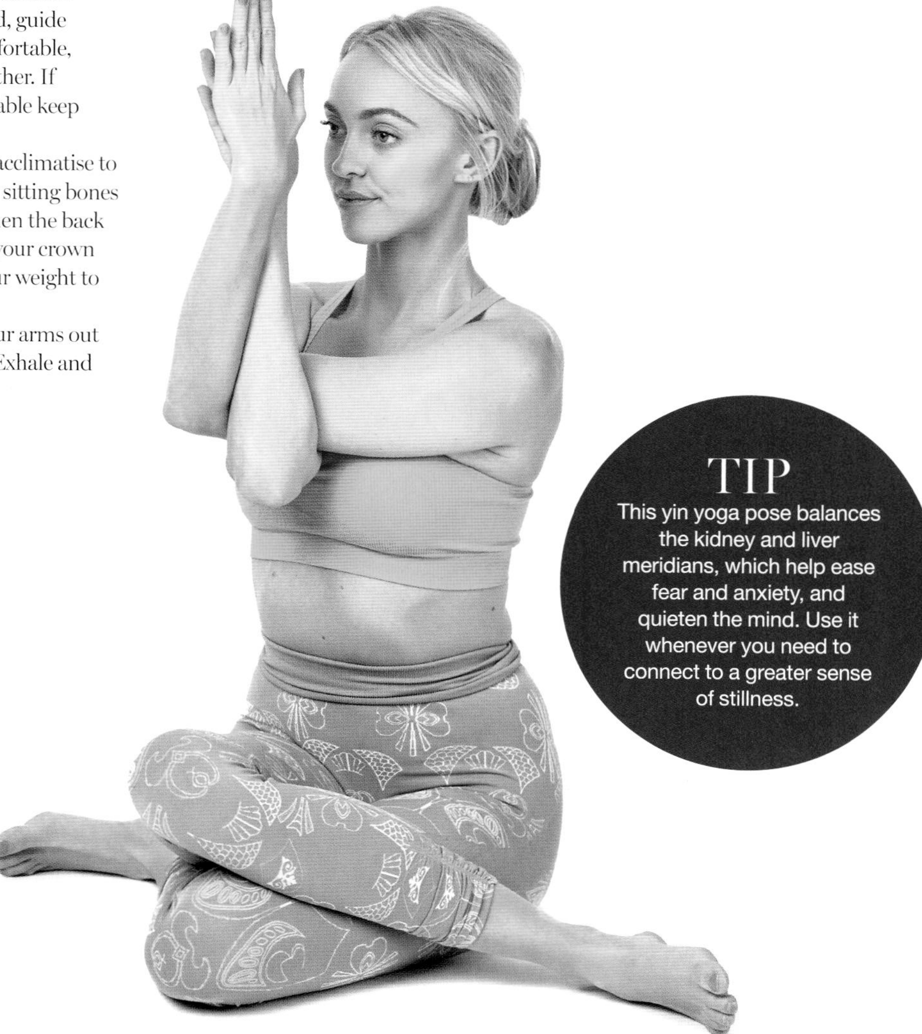

TIP

This yin yoga pose balances the kidney and liver meridians, which help ease fear and anxiety, and quieten the mind. Use it whenever you need to connect to a greater sense of stillness.

SLEEPING SWAN

- Come onto all-fours, with your hands shoulder-distance apart, about a handspan in front of your shoulders. Bring your right knee forwards and place it behind and outside your right wrist. Initially, your right shinbone may naturally rest at about a 45-degree angle, with your right heel near your left hip. As you progress, place your shin parallel to the front edge of the mat for a stronger hip opener.
- Slide your left leg straight behind you, and rest on the centre of your front thigh. Draw your left hip forward and your right hip back to square the pelvis.
- Inhale and root through your hands to lengthen your spine, extending through the crown, then, on an exhale, fold forwards over your bent leg. Place your forehead on the back of your hands or rest it on a bolster.
- This is a strong hip opener – direct your breath towards any tension in your hip to help disperse the intensity. Breathe softly and deeply for up to a minute.
- When you are ready to come out, inhale and root through your hands to come up and gently release your legs. Repeat on the other side.

GOOD FOR

- Calming
- Rests your brain
- Releases tension in your hips

TIP

If the hip of your bent leg doesn't reach the floor, place a block or folded blanket under it, so your hips are fully supported.

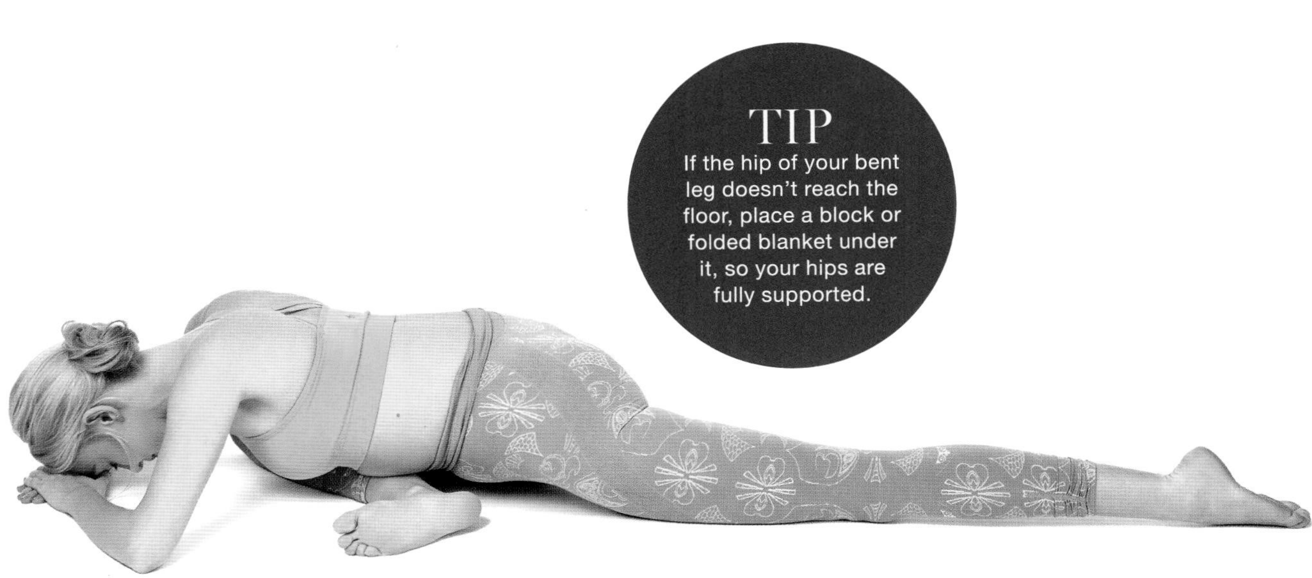

SNAIL

- Lie on your back with your knees bent, feet flat on the floor and your arms by your sides, palms down. Take a few breaths into your belly to quieten your mind.
- Bring your knees to your chest, then straighten your legs to take your feet up towards the ceiling.
- Take a deep breath in then, on an exhale, root through your hands to lift your legs up and over your head to the floor behind you, knees slightly bent, toes tucked under. At the same time, take your hands to your side ribs to support your back.
- Stay here for a few breaths, with your back slightly curved. Unlike the traditional yang pose, Plough, this yin version has a soft rounded spine. Straighten your legs and reach through your heels.
- If you are comfortable here, release your hands and extend your arms, palms facing upwards and take 10-20 slow, smooth breaths.
- To come out of the pose, raise your feet and uncurl your spine, releasing one vertebra at a time to the floor until you are flat on your back. Pause for a moment or two, then come into Bridge (p25) to realign your spine.

GOOD FOR

- Alleviates fatigue
- Calms your brain
- Eases insomnia
- Reduces stress

TIP

If your feet don't reach the floor behind you, rest them on a bolster. Alternatively, do the pose at one end of the room and let your feet rest against the wall at a comfortable height for you.

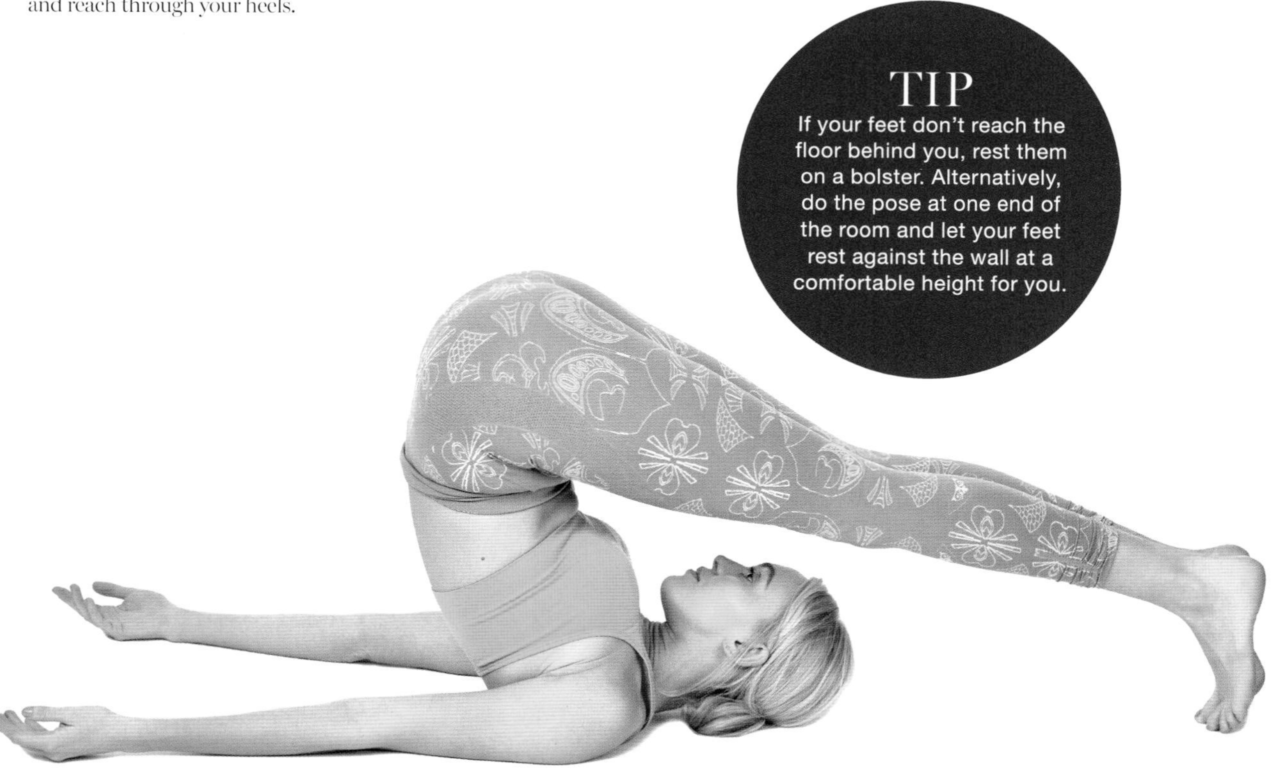

SPHINX

● Lie on your stomach with your feet shoulder-width apart, resting on the tops of your toes. Relax your buttocks and legs.
● Take your upper body weight onto your forearms, keeping them parallel, and your elbows shoulder-width apart. Spread your fingertips and root through the base of your fingers and thumbs.
● Press your weight into your forearms so you don't sink into your shoulders and draw your shoulder blades down your back. Gently engage your inner thighs, but allow your belly to sink towards the floor. Keep your neck in line with your spine and gaze softly forwards, or, if comfortable, let it reach back slightly and look upwards (A).
● Rest in the pose for three to five minutes, then lower back to the mat on an exhale.

GOOD FOR

● Tones your spine
● Stimulates your lower back
● Stimulates your thyroid (when your neck is released back)

VARIATION

SEAL (B)

● For a stronger backbend, place your hands about four inches in front of your shoulders, slightly rotated outwards, approximately the width of your mat. Keep your elbows sightly flexed and your neck in line with your spine.

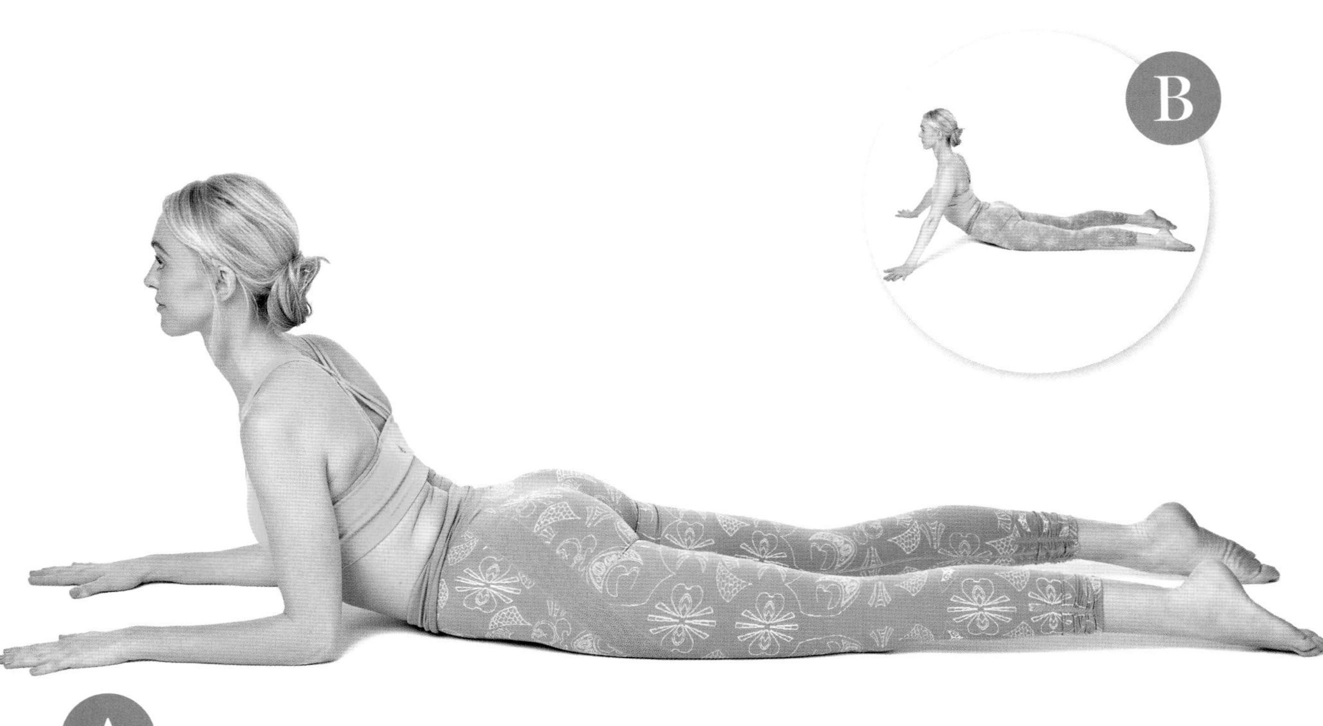

TWISTED DRAGON

● From Crescent pose (p29) with right foot forwards, heel/toe your right foot towards the right edge of your mat, then place your hands to the inside of your right foot.
● Check that your right knee is directly above your ankle, hug it into the mid-line and ground through the base of your big and little toes.
● Inhale, and gently engage your abdomen as you lift your torso and bring your hands to prayer position. On an exhale, twist to the right, hooking your left elbow outside your right thigh. Extend your heart forwards and to the right while drawing your shoulders down your back at the same time (A). Draw your navel to your spine.
● Rest in the pose for five deep breaths, before releasing on an exhale and repeating on the other side.

GOOD FOR

● Opens your hip and groin
● Releases tight hip flexors
● Strengthens the inner thigh of your front leg
● Aids digestion

VARIATION

DRAGON (B)

● Place your hands and forearms shoulder-width apart and parallel on the floor, and rest your gaze on the floor. Keep your shoulders drawing down your back and your abdomen gently engaged.

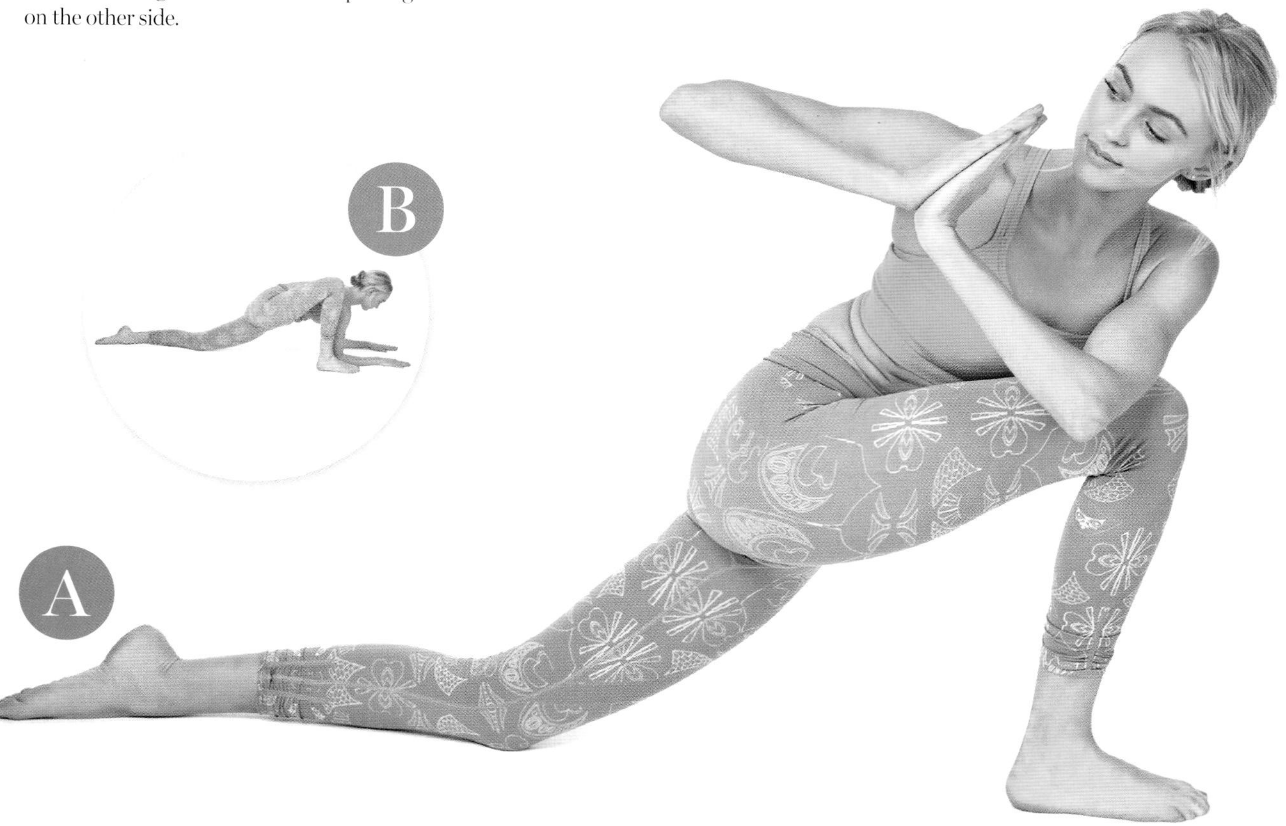

WIDE-LEGGED SEATED FORWARD FOLD

PROPS

One/two bolsters or cushions

- Sit on the floor. Take your legs wide apart, kneecaps facing the ceiling, ankles flexed, inner edges of your feet vertical and feet resting on the centre of the back of each heel. Place one or two bolsters in between your legs and place your hands on your belly, close your eyes and take three deep abdominal breaths.
- When you're ready to progress, use your hands to take the flesh of your buttocks backwards and away from your mid-line, so you can rest on the front of your sitting bones.
- Place your hands beside your hips, and root through your fingertips and sitting bones to lengthen your spine. Draw your navel to your spine, open your chest and draw your shoulder blades down your back. Float your crown up to the sky.
- When you feel ready, place your hands on the floor in front of you either side of the bolster. On an inhale, lengthen your front body by drawing your lower back forwards, then, exhale and walk your hands forwards as you fold forwards from your hips, leading with your heart.
- When you reach your edge, allow your breath to soften your body, and rest on the bolster for up to five minutes, breathing slowly and evenly, changing the direction of your head half-way through.
- To come out, inhale as you walk your hands back to bring you up to sitting.

GOOD FOR

- Deeply relaxing
- Calms your brain
- Soothes mental agitation

TIP

This can be a strong pose. If you feel a strain behind your knees, slightly bend your legs or place a folded towel under each knee.

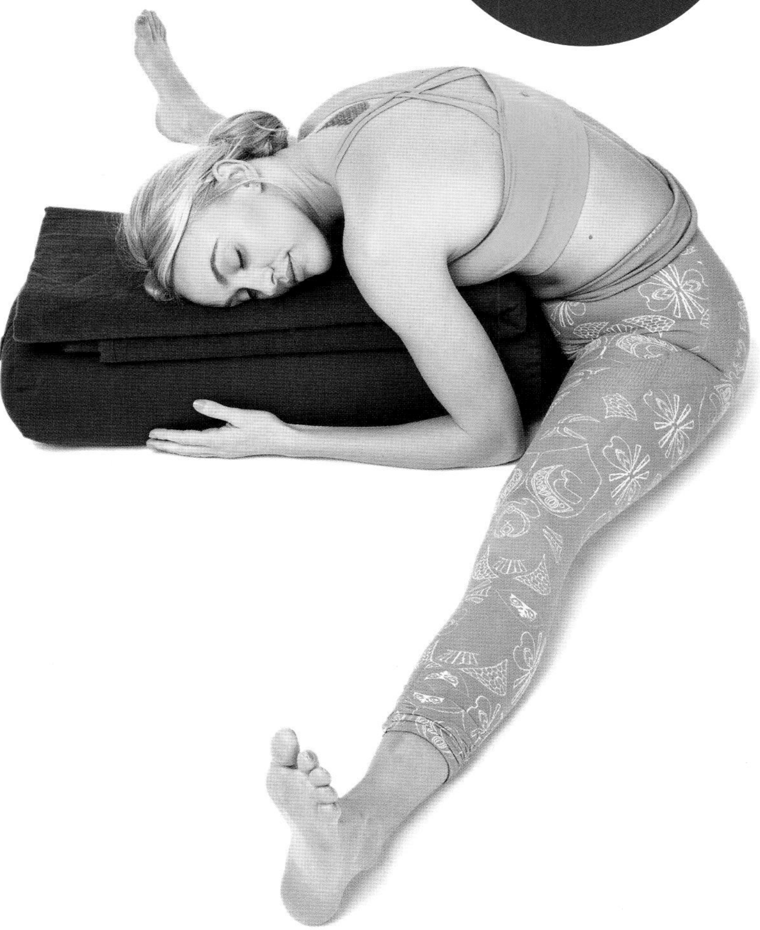

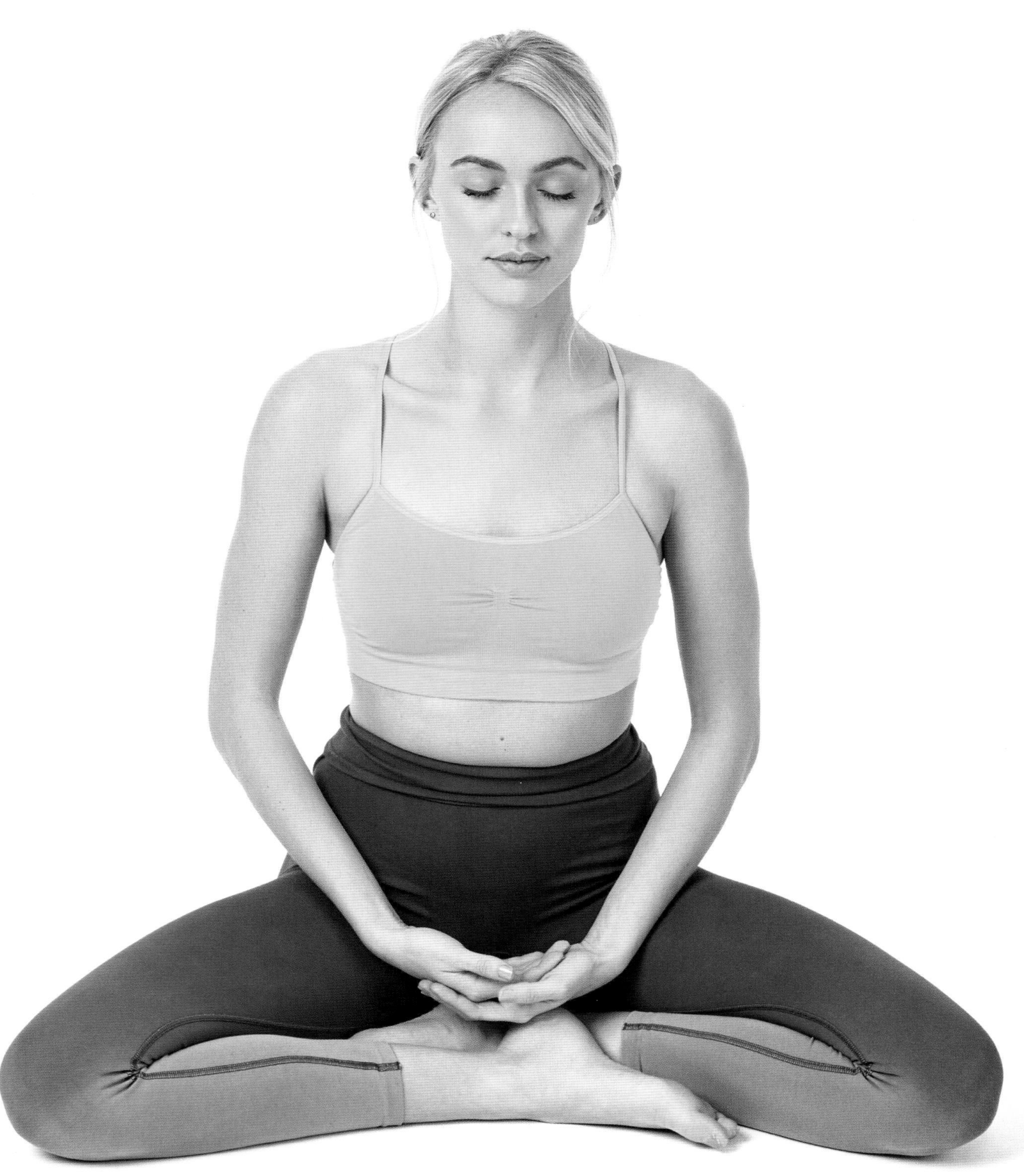

AM SEQUENCES

You've learned the main postures and have the foundations in place, so it's time to put it all together. The following sequences are designed to meet your morning goals, whether you want to ease muscle stiffness, build your strength, be focused for the day ahead or understand yourself better using mindful yoga practices. Work through the sequences slowly to familiarise yourself with the moves then, over time, you can put the book aside and focus more deeply on your experience.

AM WARM-UP POSES

CAT/COW

From all-fours, inhale, then, as you exhale, root through the base of your index fingers and thumbs and the tops of your toes as you release your head and tailbone to the floor and lift your spine towards the ceiling into Cat (A). On your next inhale, tilt your tailbone up and release your spine down into a gentle backbend. Draw your shoulders down your back, take your chest forwards and up and gently raise your head into Cow (B). Continue alternating between Cat and Cow, instigating the movement from your pelvis and following the natural pattern of your breath. Move vertebra by vertebra in a slow and fluid way.

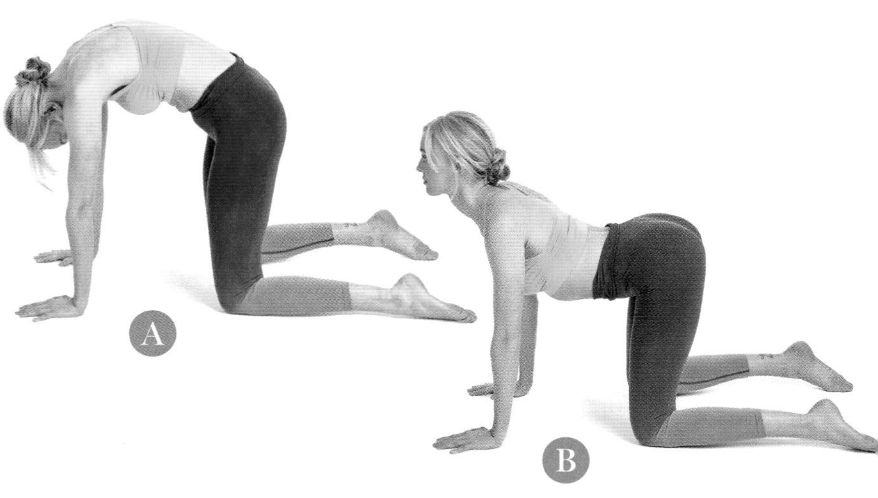

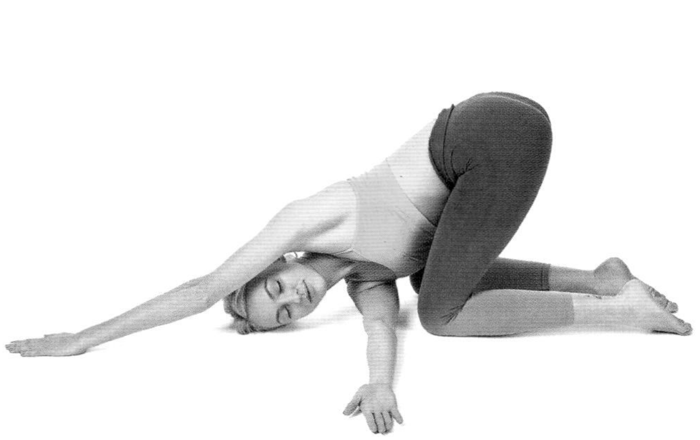

THREAD THE NEEDLE

From all-fours, with your shoulders over your wrists and hips over your knees, inhale and raise your right arm out to the side. On an exhale, slide your arm beneath your torso, palm facing up, extending your hand under your left arm and out to the side. Take your left hand forwards a few inches, then press into the floor to lift your left shoulder and deepen the twist. Exhale to release, then repeat on the other side.

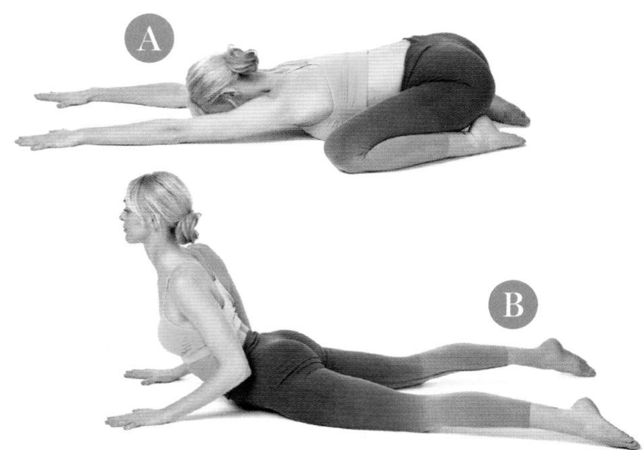

CHILD'S POSE TO COBRA

From a Wide-legged child's pose (A), inhale and root through your hands to come onto all-fours. Take your feet hip-distance apart, and exhale as you roll down the front of your body, hips leading, to lie on your stomach. With your hands beneath your shoulders, inhale and root into the floor, raising the back of your neck first, to come up into Cobra (B). On an exhale, slowly lower back to the floor. Inhale, root through your hands and lift your tailbone to come back into Child's pose (p34). Complete a few rounds, then rest in Child's pose.

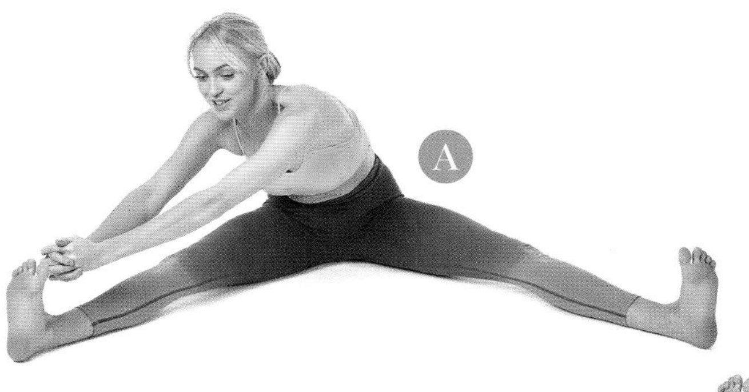

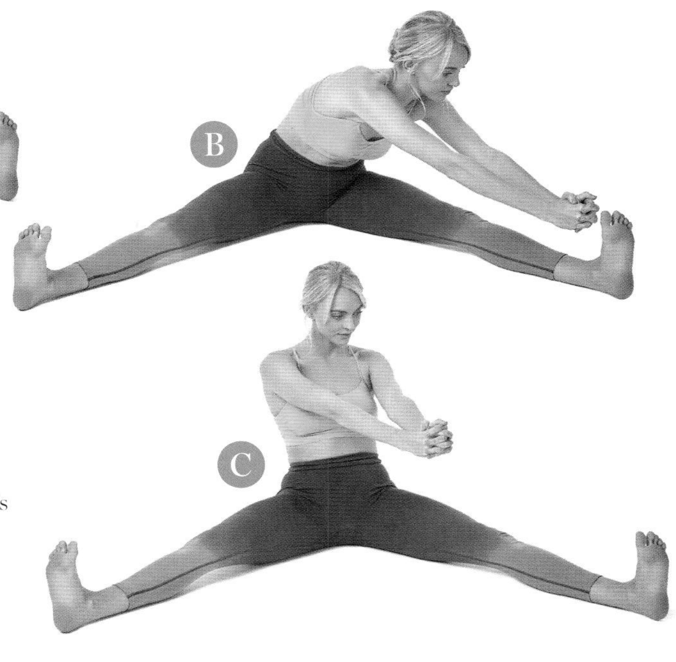

WIDE-LEGGED STIRRING THE POT

Sit on the floor with your legs wide apart. Interlace your fingers, bring your inner wrists together, and straighten your arms in front of you at chest height. On an inhale, fold forwards from your hips and, keeping your arms straight, reach your hands towards your right foot (A). Staying bent forwards, circle your arms between the centre of your feet and around to your left foot (B). As you exhale, lean backwards (C), still reaching forwards with your arms, then come forwards as your arms complete the circle at your right foot. This is one cycle. Complete five to 10 cycles, then repeat in the opposite direction.

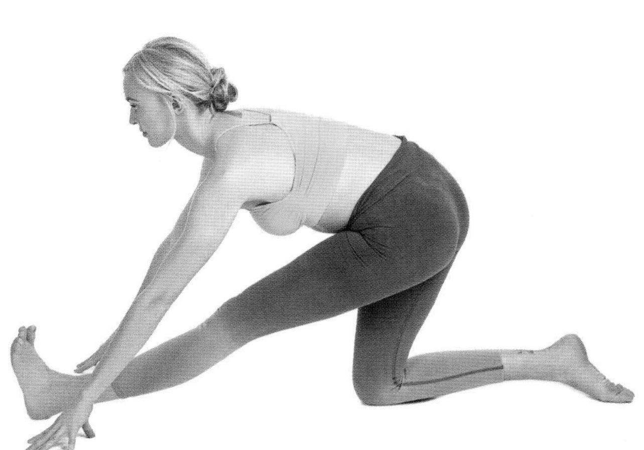

HAMSTRING STRETCH

From Lizard pose, with your right leg bent (p43), inhale and take your weight back into your hands. Lift your right hand as you heel/toe your right foot to take it a few inches towards the centre of your mat, then lower your hand again. As you exhale, reach your buttocks towards your back heel, walking your hands back as far as you need to for support. Fold forwards from your hips with a straight back and feel the stretch in your hamstrings. Take five to 10 deep breaths into the area, then rest in Child's pose (p34) before stepping your right foot forwards to repeat on the other side.

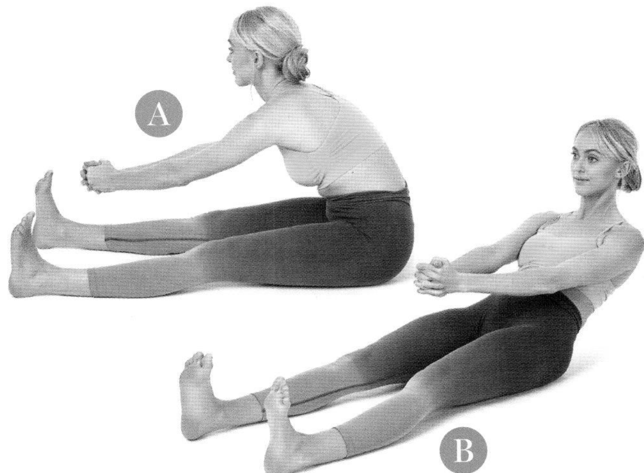

NARROW-LEGGED STIRRING THE POT

Repeat the moves for Wide-legged stirring the pot (above), this time with your legs slightly wider than hip-width apart (A) and, engaging your core, lean back as close to the mat as you are able (B). Complete five to 10 cycles, without allowing your feet to lift off the ground as you lean backwards, then repeat in the opposite direction.

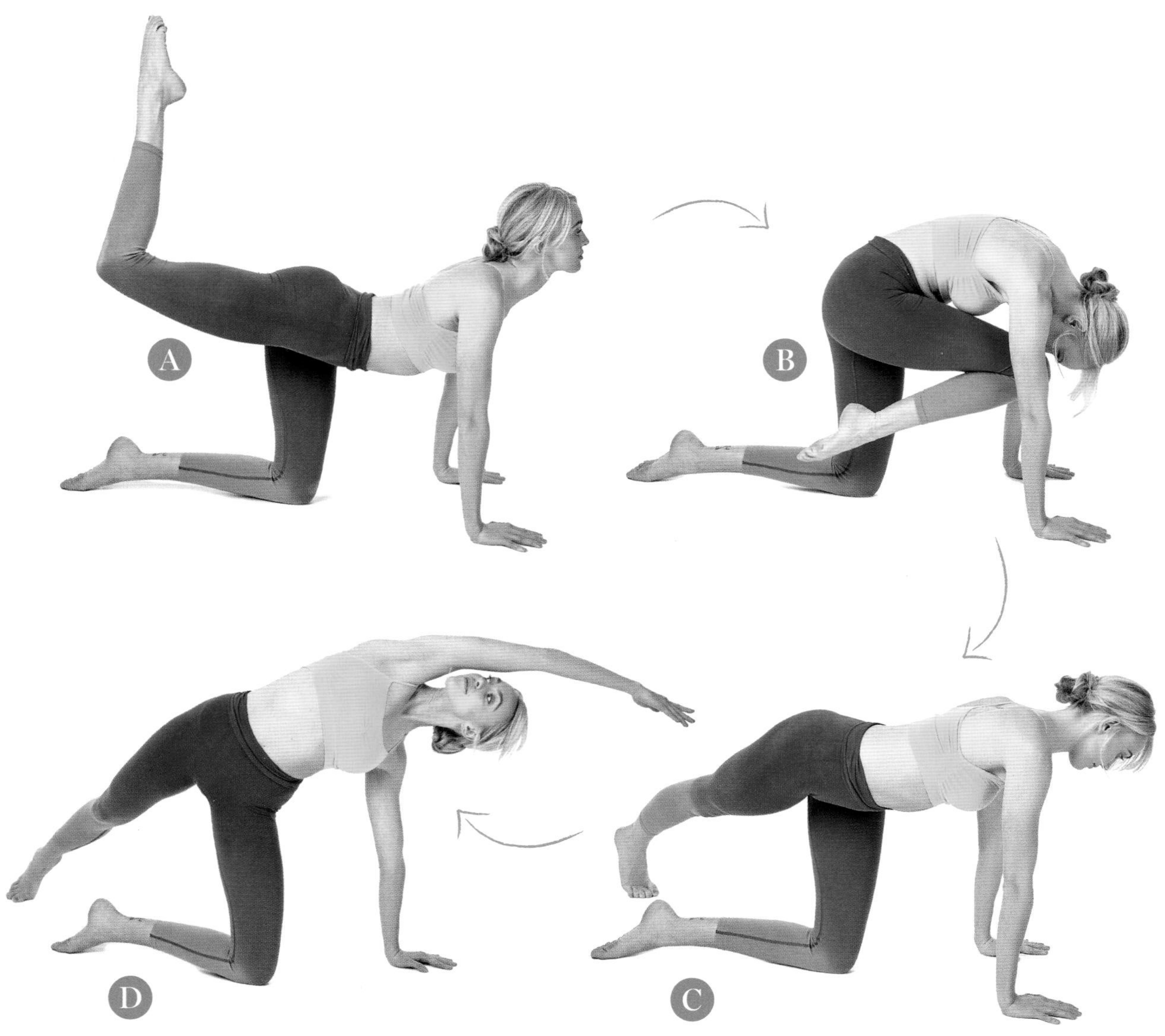

TIGER FLOW

From Cat pose (p80), inhale and stretch your right leg back and up, bending your knee and pointing your toes towards your head into Tiger (A). Pause, then, as you exhale, bring your knee towards your chest as you arc your spine upwards (B). Moving in time with your breath, repeat a few times, then, on an inhale, extend your right leg and rest your toes outside your left foot to lengthen and open the length of your right body into Side gate (C). Gaze over your left shoulder to look at your right foot.

Take a few breaths into your right ribs, then raise your right foot, place it out to the side and point your toes, keeping your left leg in the same position. Root through your left hand as you raise your right arm alongside your ear and lift into Side gate (D). Feel the stretch from your right toes all the way to your right fingertips. Take five deep breaths into your right ribs, then exhale to lower and repeat on the other side.

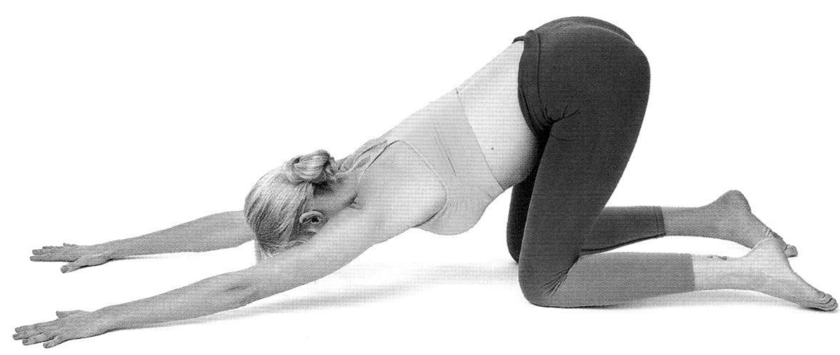

PUPPY DOG

From all-fours, with your shoulders over your wrists and hips over your knees, lie your toes flat on the floor and walk your hands forwards a hand's-length or two. Inhale, then exhale and root through your hands as you take your hips back slightly to lengthen your spine. Walk your hands forwards a few inches more, if needed, to keep your thighs vertical, then, with your arms remaining active and fingers spread, lower your head to the floor or a folded blanket. Relax your neck and take five deep breaths into your back body. To come out, release into Child's pose (p34) and rest for a moment or two.

RECLINING HAND TO TOE POSE

Lie on your back and hug your right knee in to your chest. Wrap a strap around the ball of your right foot and, on an inhale, straighten your leg. Exhale as you rotate your hip outwards and lower your leg to the side. If necessary, use your left hand to keep your left hip on the floor; otherwise extend your left arm out to the side. Beginners: if your lower back comes off the floor, bend your left knee and place your foot flat on the floor. Take five deep breaths, inhale to bring your leg back to centre and exhale to gently lower. Repeat on the other side.

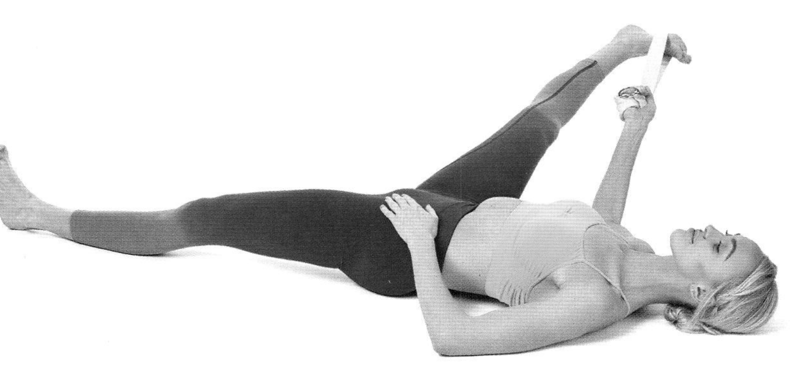

A

B

WINDSCREEN WIPERS

Come on to your back, bend your knees and rest your feet flat on the floor, ankles touching. Let your arms rest away from your body, palms facing the ceiling. Inhale, then as you exhale, let your knees float over to your left. At the same time, if comfortable for your neck, turn your head to face the right (A). Inhale back to centre, then repeat on the opposite side (B). Alternate between left and right for a few breaths to release any tension in your spine.

SUN SALUTE I

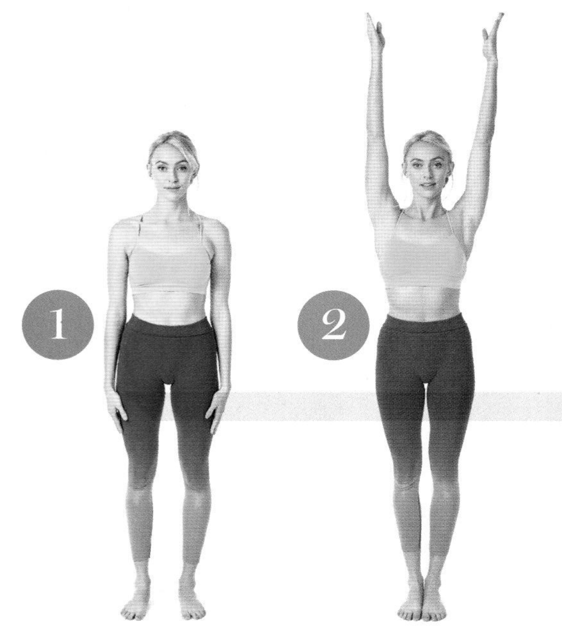

Sun salutes are a great way to wake up the body and get you moving first thing. The repeated folding and unfolding is an added benefit as it lubricates the intervertebral discs in your spine, helping to maintain their health.

Adjust the sequence according to your need, moving faster to increase your energy and strength, working slowly and mindfully to increase feelings of calm and being grounded. On the first round, take three to five breaths in each pose to focus on good alignment and to give your body time to acclimatise to the pose. On subsequent rounds, flow freely from one posture to the next, following the breathing pattern below. Link each movement to your breath, breathing into your belly or using Ocean breath (p98).

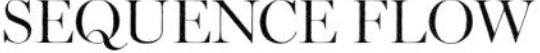

SEQUENCE FLOW

● 1 MOUNTAIN POSE
p44
Inhale, root through your feet and take your arms out to the sides and overhead to...

● 2 EXTENDED MOUNTAIN POSE
p44
Exhale and take your arms to the sides and down into...

● 3 STANDING FORWARD FOLD
p52
Inhale as you step your right leg back to...

● 4 CRESCENT
p29
Exhale and step your left leg back to...

● 5 DOWNWARD DOG
p30
Take five deep breaths here, 'walking the dog' by bending one knee then the other, and focus on lifting your tailbone up and back to lengthen your spine.

● 6 CATERPILLAR
Pause your breath as you lower your knees and chest to the floor, and then your abdomen. Then inhale into...

● 7 COBRA
p28
Exhale and root through your hands to lift back into...

● 8 DOWNWARD DOG
Inhale as you step your right foot forwards into...

● 9 CRESCENT
Exhale and step your left foot forwards into...

● 10 STANDING FORWARD FOLD
Inhale, taking your arms out to the side and overhead to...

● 11 EXTENDED MOUNTAIN POSE
Exhale your arms out to the side and to prayer, back into...

● 12 MOUNTAIN POSE
Repeat, leading with your left leg. This forms one round.

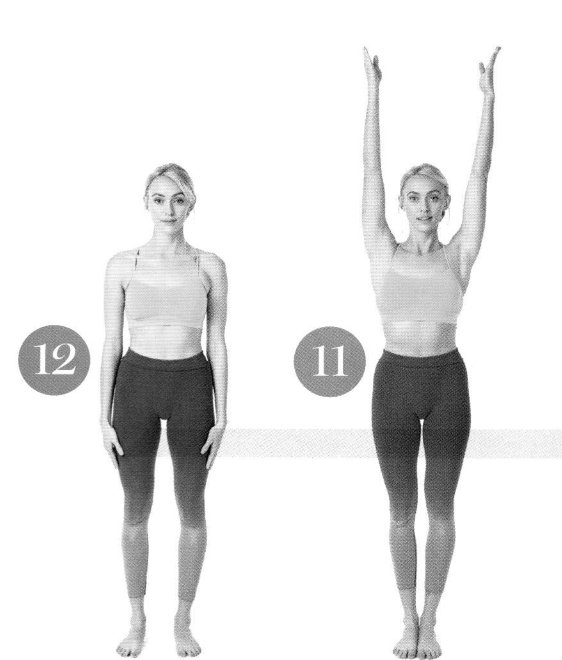

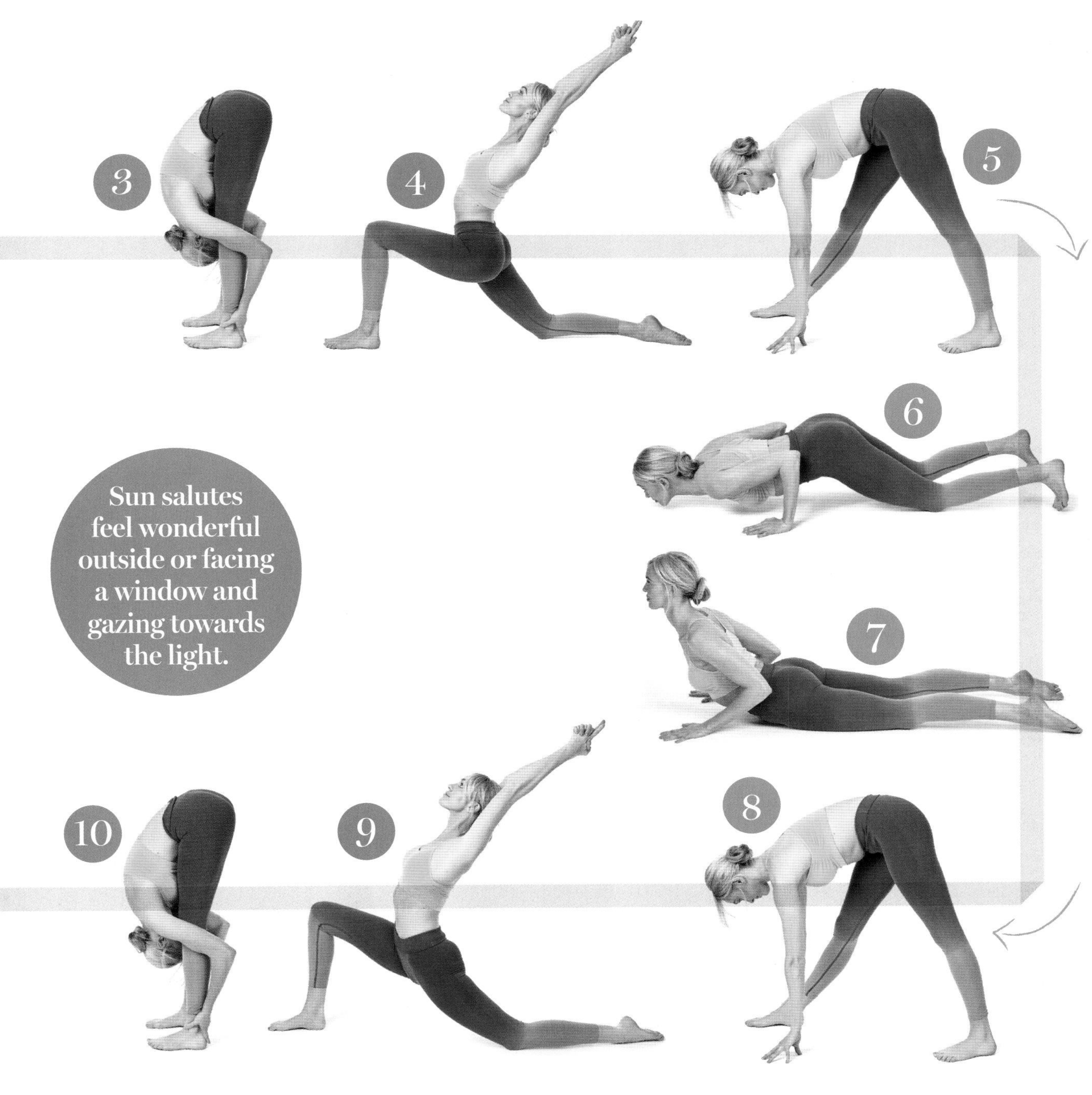

Sun salutes feel wonderful outside or facing a window and gazing towards the light.

SUN SALUTE II

This is a more challenging Sun salute, based on the Ashtanga Intermediate Series. Use this sequence when you want to build your strength and boost your energy, using Ocean breath (p98). Start with three rounds and build up as your strength grows.

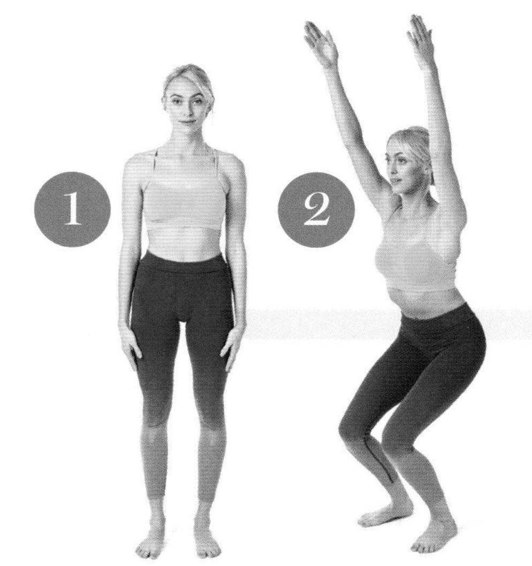

SEQUENCE FLOW

● 1 MOUNTAIN POSE
p44
Inhale, root through your feet and take your arms overhead into...

● 2 CHAIR
p27
Exhale, straighten your legs and hinge from your hips into...

● 3 STANDING FORWARD FOLD
p52
Inhale and extend your spine into...

● 4 HALF STANDING FORWARD FOLD
p52
Exhale and step or jump back into...

● 5 PUSH-UP
Inhale to...

● 6 COBRA
p28
Exhale and lift your buttocks into...

● 7 DOWNWARD DOG
p30
Inhale and step your left foot forwards into...

● 8 HIGH LUNGE
p41
Exhale, lower your hands and step back into...

● 9 PUSH-UP
Inhale into...

● 10 COBRA
Exhale and lift your buttocks into...

● 11 DOWNWARD DOG
Inhale and step your right foot forwards into ...

● 12 HIGH LUNGE
Exhale and bring your right leg back into...

● 13 PUSH-UP
Inhale into...

● 14 COBRA
Exhale and lift your buttocks into...

● 15 DOWNWARD DOG
Inhale and step or jump forwards into...

● 16 HALF STANDING FORWARD FOLD
Exhale into...

● 17 STANDING FORWARD FOLD
Inhale and come back up into...

● 18 CHAIR
Exhale and straighten your legs to return to...

● 19 MOUNTAIN POSE

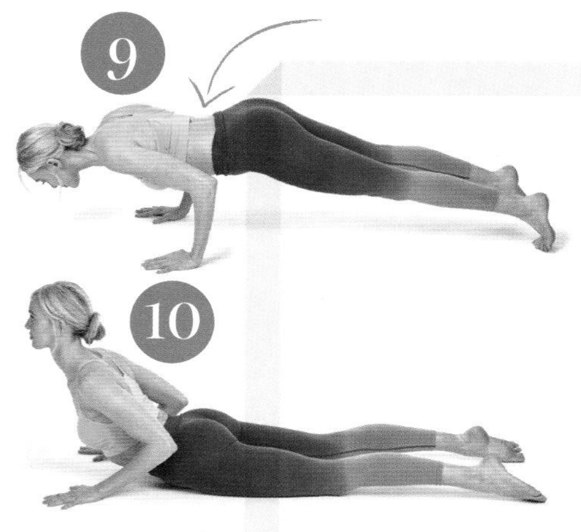

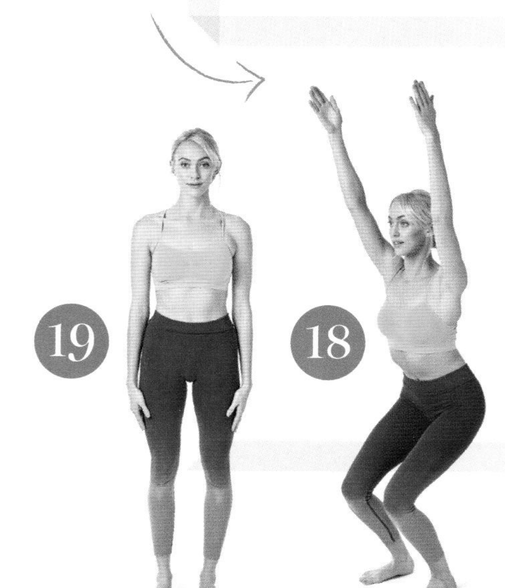

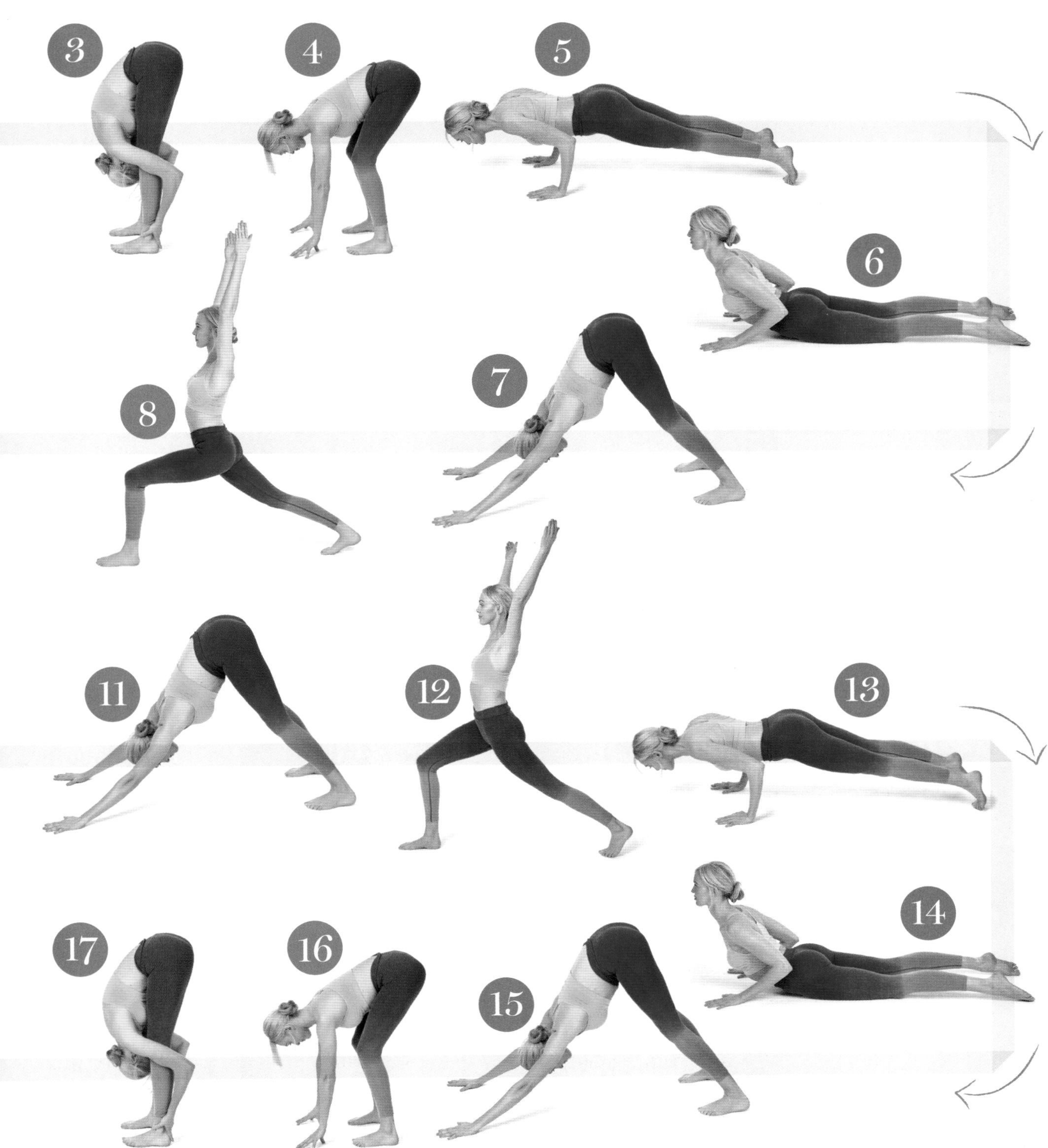
3
4
5
6
8
7
11
12
13
17
16
15
14

MORNING REFRESHER

If you wake up feeling groggy – either from a late night, poor sleep or simply because you've been working too hard – an energising yoga sequence first thing can prepare you physically and mentally for the challenges of the day ahead. This sequence includes lots of inversions, where your head is below your heart, to encourage blood flow to your brain. Flooding your brain with fresh oxygen will leave you refreshed and energised, while the chest openers bring a feeling of expansion to your system. For an extra energising boost, lightly jump back into Plank and forwards from Downward dog in the Sun salute.

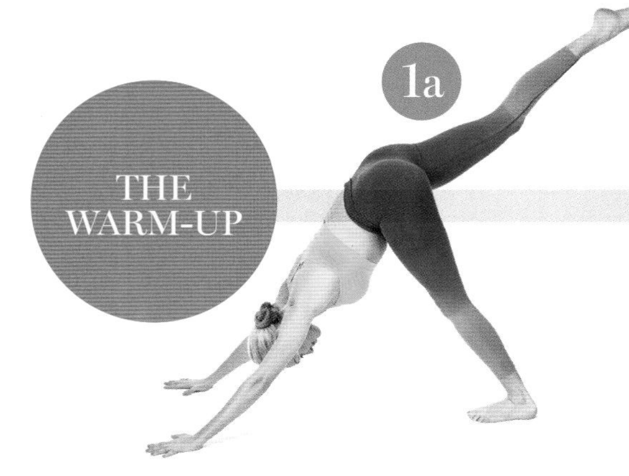

THE WARM-UP

A CAT/COW
p80
Flow between the two poses for several breaths.

B TIGER
p82
Right side. Flow between the two poses for several breaths then, with your right leg raised, move straight into...

C SIDE STRETCH
p33

D SIDE GATE
p82

Repeat poses B-D with your left leg.

E HERO TWIST
p40

SUN SALUTE II
p86

THE SEQUENCE

1a & 1b DOWNWARD DOG SPLITS
p31
Right side. Flow between the two poses for several breaths, then with your right leg raised, step your right foot forwards into...

2 HIGH LUNGE
p41
Straighten your right leg and lower your right arm into...

3 TRIANGLE
p55
Place your right hand on the floor a foot in front of you and lift your left leg into...

4 HALF MOON
p38
Swivel on your feet to face the opposite direction.

Lower your leg and repeat poses 1-4 with your left leg.

5 WIDE-LEGGED STANDING FORWARD FOLD
p59

6 DOLPHIN
p30

7 SUPPORTED HEADSTAND*
p53
Beginners, perform against a wall or do Legs up the wall (p42).

8 DOWNWARD DOG
p30

9 HERO
p40.

TO FINISH

If you have time, do a few rounds of Bellows breath (p99), then rest with your eyes closed, and allow your breathing to return to normal.

* Replace Headstand with Legs up the wall (p42), if you have your period.

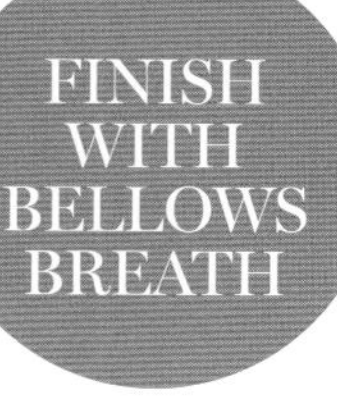

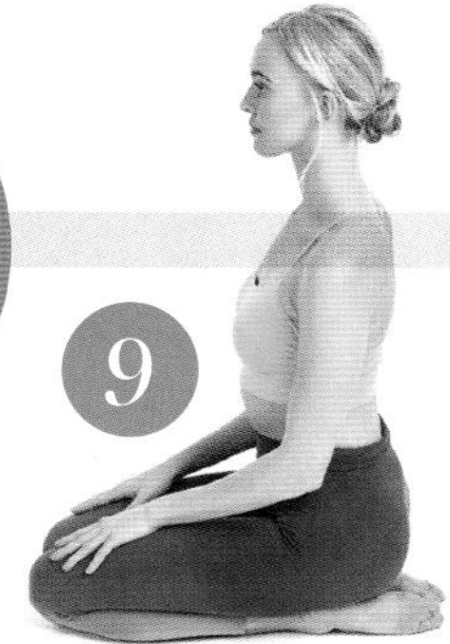

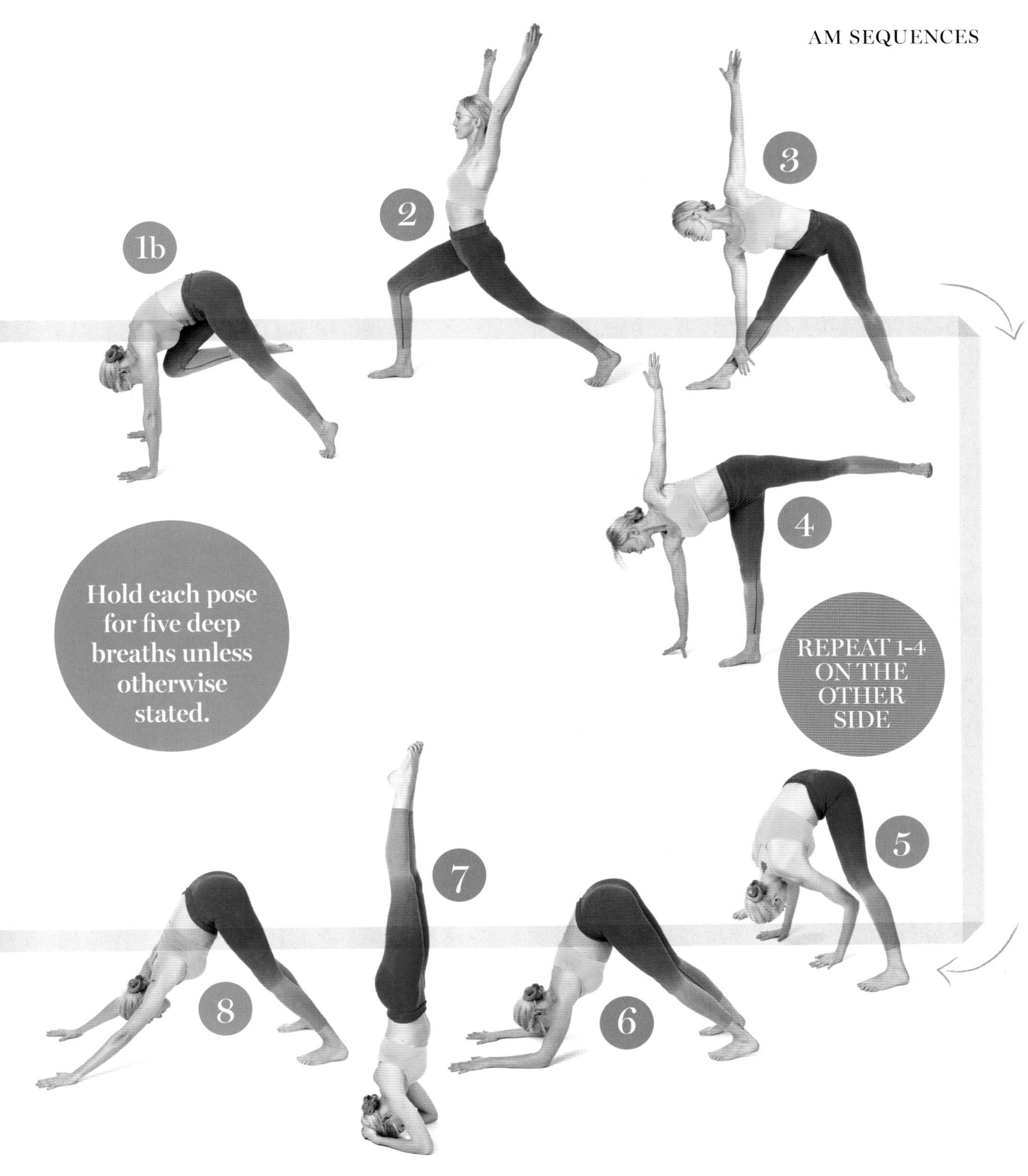
1b
2
3
4
Hold each pose for five deep breaths unless otherwise stated.
REPEAT 1-4 ON THE OTHER SIDE
5
7
8
6

BUILD YOUR STRENGTH

When you want to develop more muscle strength, aim for shorter sessions more frequently rather than one long session once a week. Try this sequence two or three times a week, interspersing it with the Stretch sequence (p92). The Plank poses work your upper body and, along with the Boat pose, build a stronger core, while the dynamic lunges challenge your quads. Balances constantly work the stabilising muscles in your legs and feet as well as your abdominals – focusing on a point in front of you will help you to stay stable. If the sequence feels too challenging, simply hold the poses for less time or do fewer repetitions, increasing the duration as your strength builds. If the sequence feels too easy, increase the duration or reps.

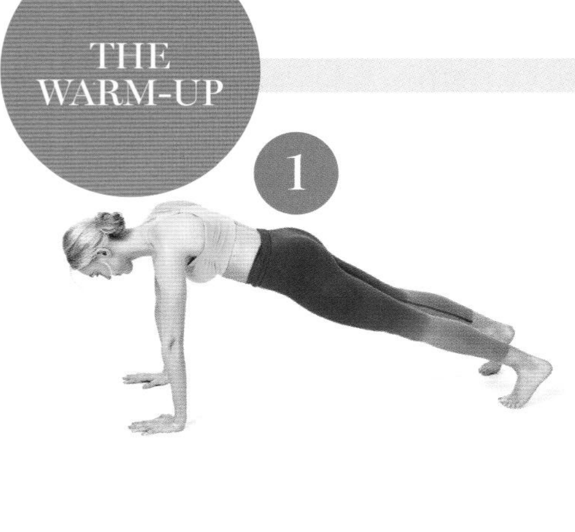

THE WARM-UP

A EASY POSE TWIST
p33

B EASY POSE SIDE STRETCH
p33

C WIDE-LEGGED STIRRING THE POT
p59
Move five to 10 times clockwise and five to 10 times anticlockwise.

D NARROW-LEGGED STIRRING THE POT
p59
Move five to 10 times clockwise and five to 10 times anticlockwise.

E HERO WITH BACKBEND
p40

SUN SALUTE II
p86

THE SEQUENCE

1 PLANK
p46
Hold for up to one minute.

2 SIDE PLANK
p46
Hold for 30 seconds then repeat on the other side. Lower back into plank, then step forward into...

3 DYNAMIC HIGH LUNGE
p41
Circle both arms five to 10 times clockwise and five to 10 times anticlockwise. Lower your arms on an exhale as you simultaneously lower your back knee. Inhale as your arms circle back up, straightening your back leg at the same time. Pause, then, when you are ready, take your weight onto your front foot and raise your back leg into...

4 WARRIOR III
p57
Lower your right arm and open your chest to the side to come into...

5 HALF MOON
p38

Repeat poses 3-5 on the other side.

6 GARLAND
p36

7 BOAT
p24

8 BRIDGE WITH RAISED LEG
p25
Hold for 30-60 seconds on each leg.

9 RECLINING TWIST
p48.

TO FINISH

Rest in Relaxation pose (p49) for five to 10 minutes, allowing your breath and heart rate to settle and your mind to become still once more.

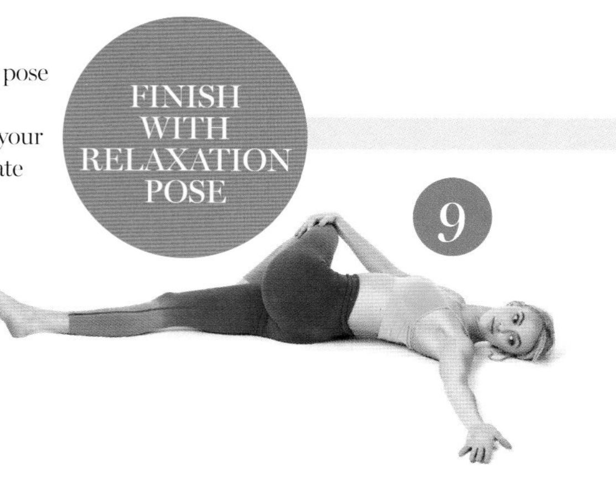

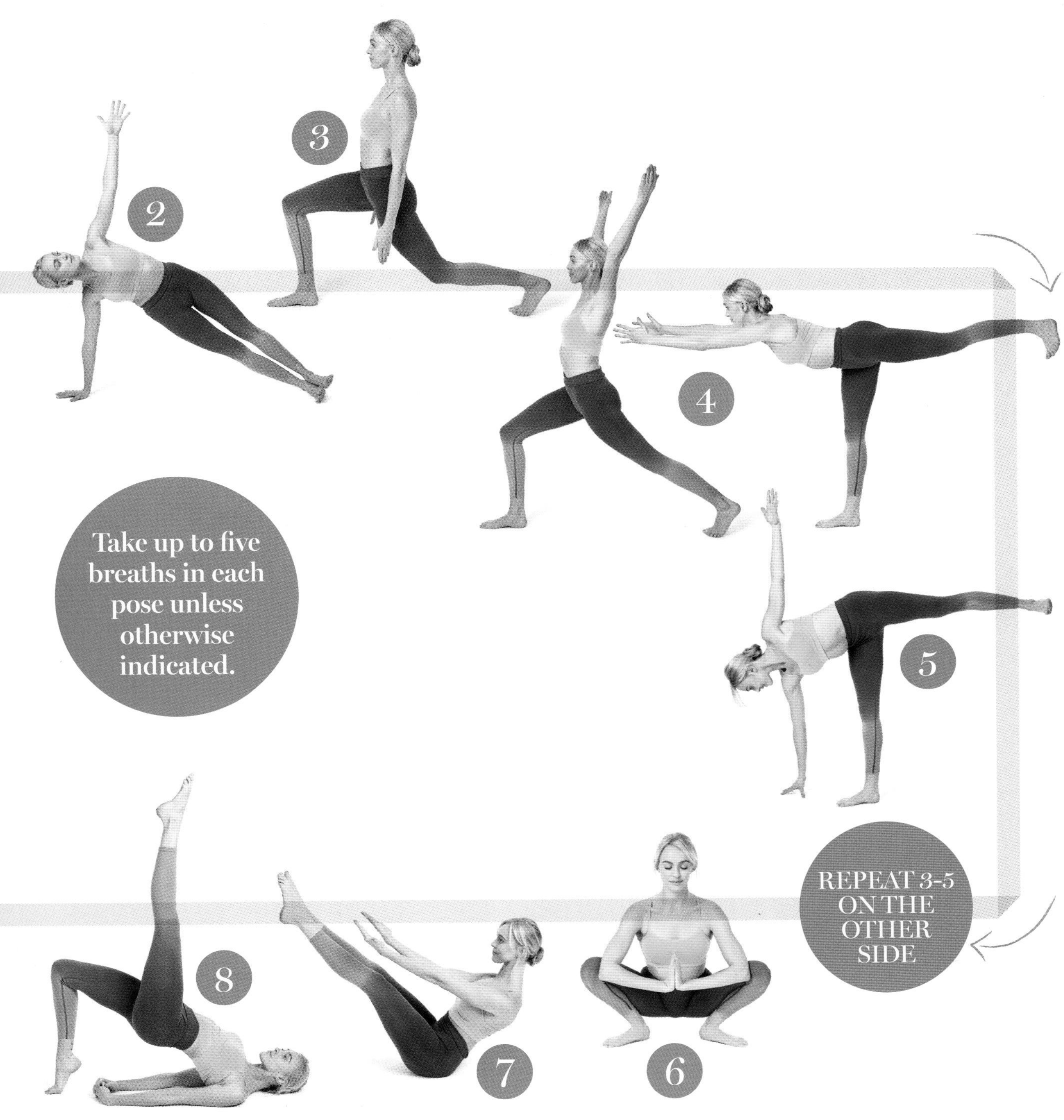
2
3
4
5
6
7
8
Take up to five breaths in each pose unless otherwise indicated.
REPEAT 3-5 ON THE OTHER SIDE

GENTLE STRETCH

If you've not had a good night's sleep, a gentle sequence is the perfect way to ease your mind and body into the day ahead. This sequence will mobilise your spine in three planes of movement – forwards, backwards and sideways – and incorporate twists to bring a sense of fluidity to your body after sleep. The hip openers, quad and hamstring stretches and shoulder releases work your major muscle groups and leave you feeling gently energised.

THE WARM-UP

1

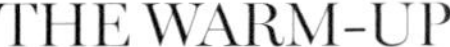

THE WARM-UP

A EXTENDED CHILD'S POSE WITH SIDE STRETCH
p34

B THREAD THE NEEDLE
p80

C EXTENDED CHILD'S POSE TO COBRA
p34 and p28
Flow between both poses.

D DOWNWARD DOG
p30
Reach alternative heels towards the ground, then walk your feet to your hands to come into...

E STANDING FORWARD FOLD
p52
Sway gently from side to side, then slowly uncurl your spine to come up to standing and roll your shoulders up, back and down five times.

SUN SALUTE I
p84
Do 1-3 rounds.

THE SEQUENCE

1 MOUNTAIN POSE WITH EAGLE ARMS
p44 and p32

2 CHAIR TWIST p27

3 WIDE-LEGGED STANDING FORWARD FOLD
p59
Reach your hands to your right leg and then your left.

4 WIDE-LEGGED STANDING FORWARD FOLD, ARMS FORWARD
p59
Pivot on your right foot to come into...

5 CRESCENT MOON p29
Lower your arms and place your forearms inside your left foot then raise your right knee to come into...

6 LIZARD p43
Lower your right knee, place one hand either side of your front foot and take your tailbone back to come into...

7 HAMSTRING STRETCH
p81
Bring your hands beneath your shoulders, extend your left foot behind you and outside your right foot to come into...

8 SIDE GATE p82
Come back to all fours.

Repeat poses 5-8 on your other leg.

9 HERO, WITH BACKBEND
p40.

TO FINISH

Pause for a couple of breaths in Extended child pose (p34), then come onto your back, take your arms overhead and stretch from your fingertips to your toes. Rest for five minutes in Relaxation pose (p49), sensing how your body feels now.

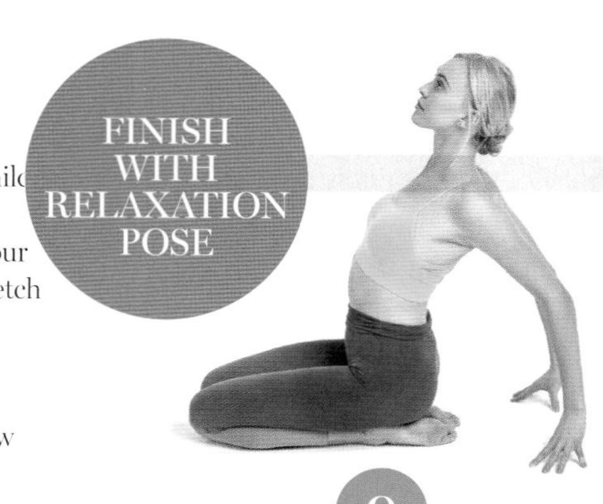

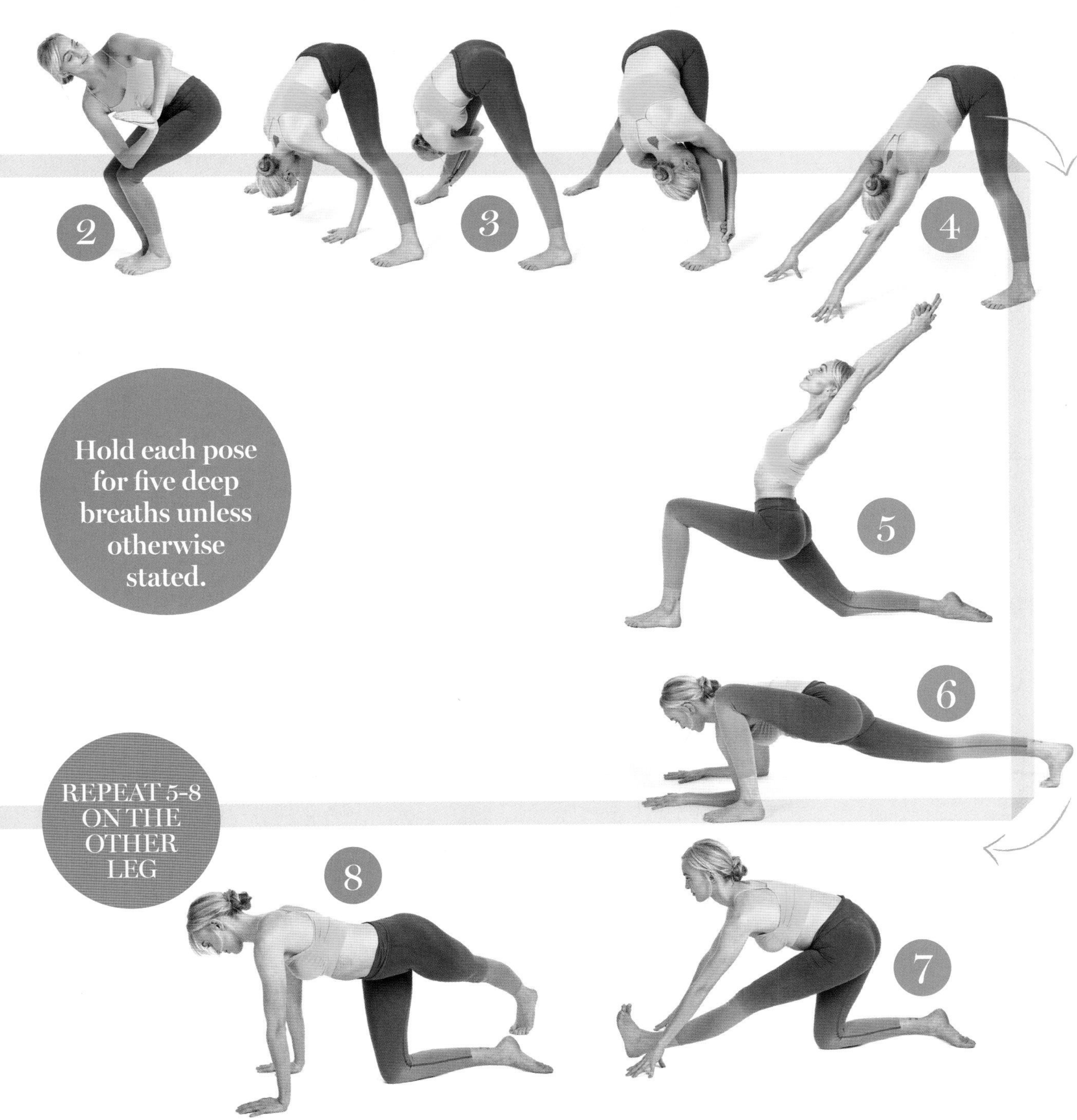
2
3
4
5
6
7
8
Hold each pose for five deep breaths unless otherwise stated.
REPEAT 5-8 ON THE OTHER LEG

FIND YOUR FOCUS

A busy or scattered mind can make it hard to concentrate, not just on the task ahead, but also on what you need to do to create the life you want. Fortunately, research published in the *Journal of Physical Activity & Health* shows that just 20 minutes of yoga a day can help to sharpen your mind. Balance poses are the ideal way to hone your focus, while Warrior II, the arm position in particular, teaches you to channel your energy in a single direction.

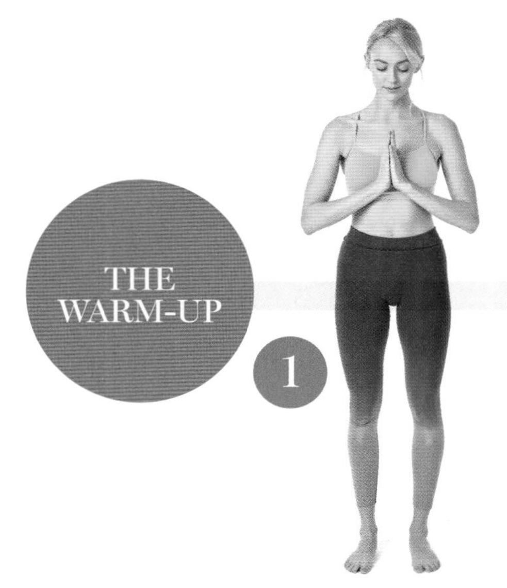

THE WARM-UP

A EASY POSE
p33
Practise Alternate nostril breathing (p123) for five minutes.

B EASY SIDE STRETCH
p33

C EASY TWIST
p33

D CAT/COW
p80

E LYING EXTENDED HAND TO TOE POSE
Hug your knee into your chest for a couple of breaths before extending out to the side, using a strap if needed.

SUN SALUTE I
p84
Do three rounds.

THE SEQUENCE

1 MOUNTAIN POSE, PRAYER HANDS
p44

2 WARRIOR II
p56
Perform on both sides, then move on to...

3 EAGLE
p32
Perform on both sides, then move on to...

4 EXTENDED HAND TO TOE POSE
p35
Perform on both sides, then move on to...

5 GARLAND
p36

6 SEATED FORWARD FOLD
p50

7 BOAT
p24

8 COBRA
p28

9 HERO TWIST
p40.

TO FINISH

Rest in Hero, or any comfortable seated pose. If you have time do the meditation on p100-101, if you only have 20 minutes, just do Part II.

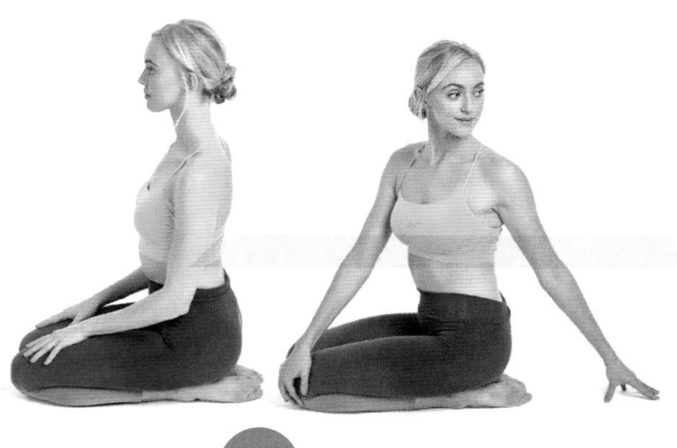

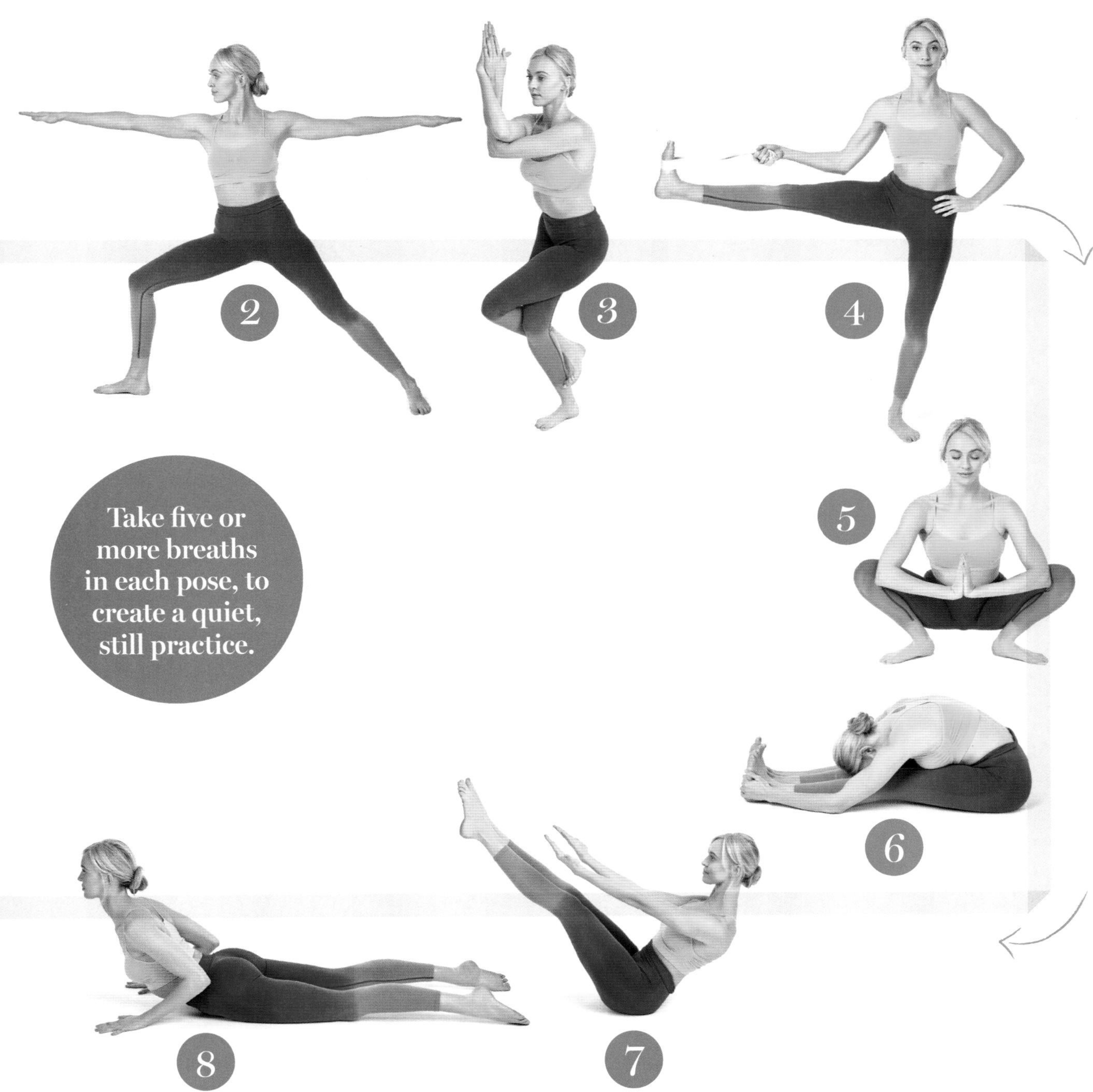

Take five or more breaths in each pose, to create a quiet, still practice.

MINDFUL MORNING

The practice of mindful yoga is slightly different from other types in that, rather than closely following instructions or trying to remember what you've previously been told about a posture, you listen to your body, moment by moment, paying particular attention to the physical sensations, emotions and thoughts you are experiencing. Treating yourself with kindness and acceptance, move at your own pace and tune in to the wisdom of your body to find your own version of the pose - one that most supports how you are in this given moment. Aim for a slow, reflective practice and stay very present with your breath, returning to it each time your mind wanders off. This sequence invites you to practise with your eyes closed, so you can turn deeply inwards.

TIP

Follow your instincts, particularly as you transition between poses. Feel free to move your body in the way that feels right for you, adding in an extra stretch or returning to Mountain (p44) or Child's pose (p34) in between each posture to check-in with your body/mind, using the Mindful meditation (33)as a template. As you become more experienced with this way of practising you may like to design your own sequence, tuning into your body after each pose and deciding what your body needs next. If you need some suggestions, look through the poses section (p24-p77) and begin with three standing poses, followed by two seated poses.

THE WARM-UP

A RELAXATION POSE – PRANAYAMA, FULL YOGIC BREATH (FIVE MINUTES)
p122

B FREE MOVEMENT (FIVE MINUTES)
Still in Relaxation pose, tune in to how your body feels now, and bring gentle movement to areas that you feel would benefit from it. For example, drawing your knees to your chest, rocking on your back, twisting to your side, circling your ankles or wrists, extending your arms overhead. When you feel ready, come up to sit in...

C EASY POSE – MINDFUL MEDITATION (FIVE MINUTES)
p33

D SET AN INTENTION FOR YOUR PRACTICE (THREE MINUTES)
p15

E EASY SIDE STRETCH
p33

F CAT/COW
p80
Again, experiment with free movement, maybe swaying your hips from side to side, or bending alternate elbows and rolling through your shoulders.

THE SEQUENCE

1 CLOSED EYE MOUNTAIN POSE (THREE TO FIVE MINUTES)
p44
Start with your hands by your sides. Notice how it feels to be standing. How is your weight distributed? What sensations do you notice in your body? There's nothing you need to change, unless it feels nourishing to do so, just be aware of what you're feeling and accept it with kindness. When you feel ready, take your hands to prayer position, and become aware of the difference this makes to your experience.

2 WARRIOR II (TWO TO THREE MINUTES)
p56
In this pose, notice how it feels to do a strong posture, really working your muscles. After a few moments, soften your muscles and try a gentle version of the pose. Which do you prefer today? Try the posture with your eyes open and with them closed. What difference does it make, and which nourishes you most?

3 WIDE-LEGGED STANDING FORWARD FOLD OR DOWNWARD DOG (TWO TO THREE MINUTES)
p59 and p30
Tune into your body and sense which of these poses feels best for you today. If you need to, try both, then choose the one that feels right. Spend a minute or two in free movement, moving your hips or shoulders to explore what feels good, then settle into stillness for a few minutes, noticing how your body/mind is responding.

4 CAMEL (ONE TO TWO MINUTES)
p26
This is a strong heart-opening pose. Don't push yourself, but move into it gently, only going as far back as feels comfortable – notice how you feel as you do so. You may find you become more aware of any emotions you may be feeling. Accept them with kindness. If the pose feels too strong, do Hero with backbend (p40) instead.

5 CHILD'S POSE (THREE TO FIVE MINUTES)
p34
Rest in the pose, allowing everything to settle, and simply notice how you feel after your Mindful yoga practice.

TO FINISH

If you have time, come to a comfortable seated position and do Part II of the meditation on p100-101.

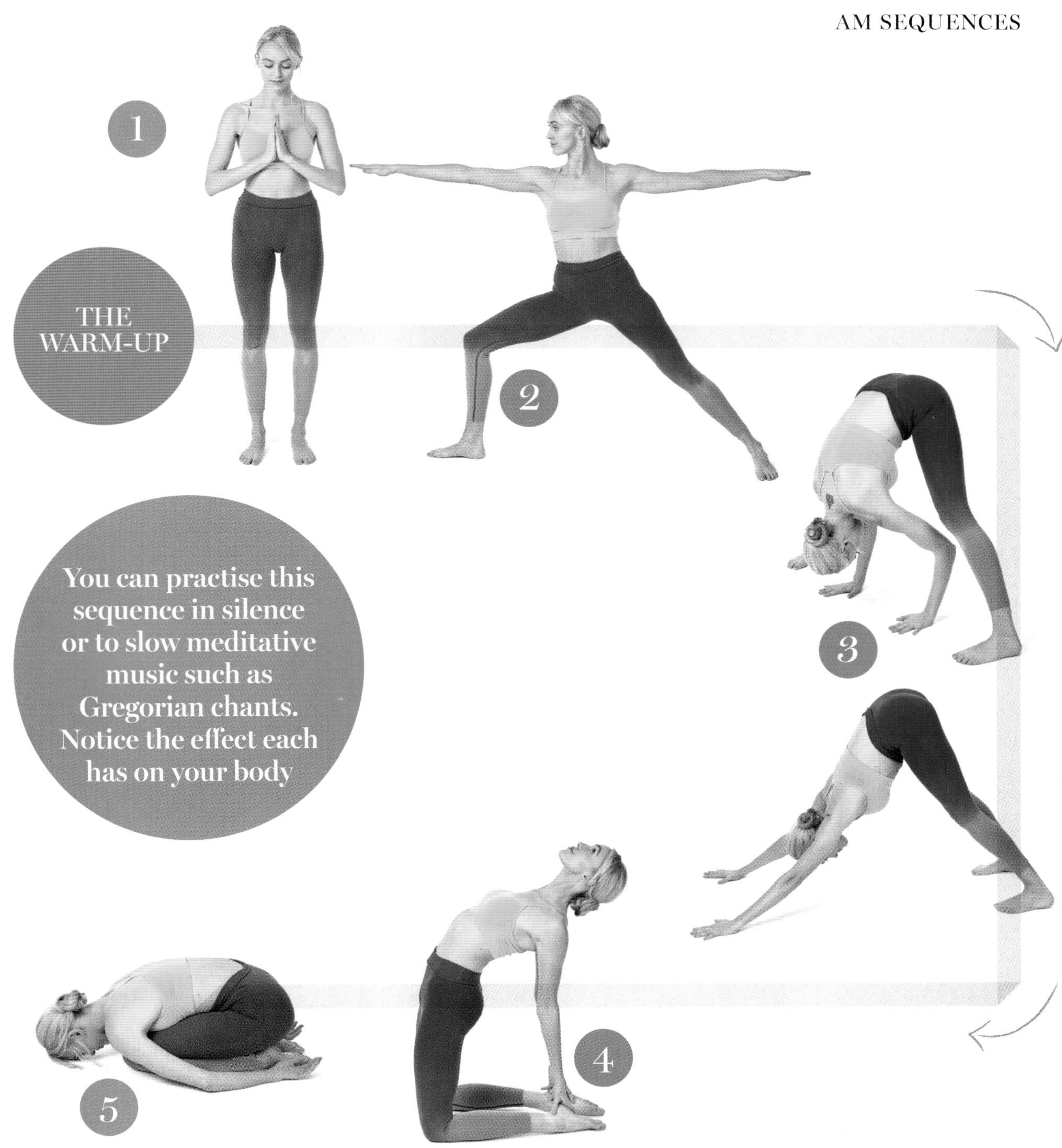
1
THE WARM-UP
2
3
You can practise this sequence in silence or to slow meditative music such as Gregorian chants. Notice the effect each has on your body
4
5

OCEAN BREATH
UJJAYI

In yoga, you can tailor your breathing to suit your needs by choosing a strong, fast breath when you want to feel energised and a slow, deep breathing pattern when you want to calm your mind and reduce tension.

Ujjayi breathing works on every cell in your body. Use it when you are doing an uplifting yoga practice to boost your energy and focus your mind.

- Begin in Relaxation pose (p49) and spend a few moments allowing your mind to start slowing down and your breathing to settle into a natural, slightly slower, rhythm.
- Gently close your eyes and gradually deepen your breathing, inhaling to a count of three and exhaling to a count of six. As this pattern becomes established, bring your attention to the pause period after the exhale and allow it to naturally lengthen. Consciously release any tension as you exhale, letting your body soften and sink deeper into the mat.
- After a few moments, let your breathing return to normal then, on your next inhalation, imagine a fine golden thread of light filtering down from the sky and entering the front of your throat. Sense it travel to the back of your throat, then, as you exhale, feel the light float up from the back of your throat to the front and up towards the sky again.
- Continue to visualise this golden light and, with each breath, sense it entering and leaving your throat. This will naturally encourage your breath to slow down. Be here for a few minutes, allowing a softness and stillness to settle around you.
- When you feel ready, slowly and mindfully come up to a comfortable seated position, sitting on a block or bolster if your back rounds.
- Become still once more, then continue drawing a thread of golden light towards your throat, this time from the horizon rather than the sky. Let a sense of quietness envelop you for a few more moments, then gently let your breath return to normal.
- Finally, gently open your lips and breathe in and out through your mouth, this time making a soft 'haaa' sound as you do. This will slightly close your throat, the key action of Ocean breath.
- Continue for a few more moments, breathing gently, so that only someone sitting close to your would hear the 'haa' sound, then gently let it go and softly open your eyes.

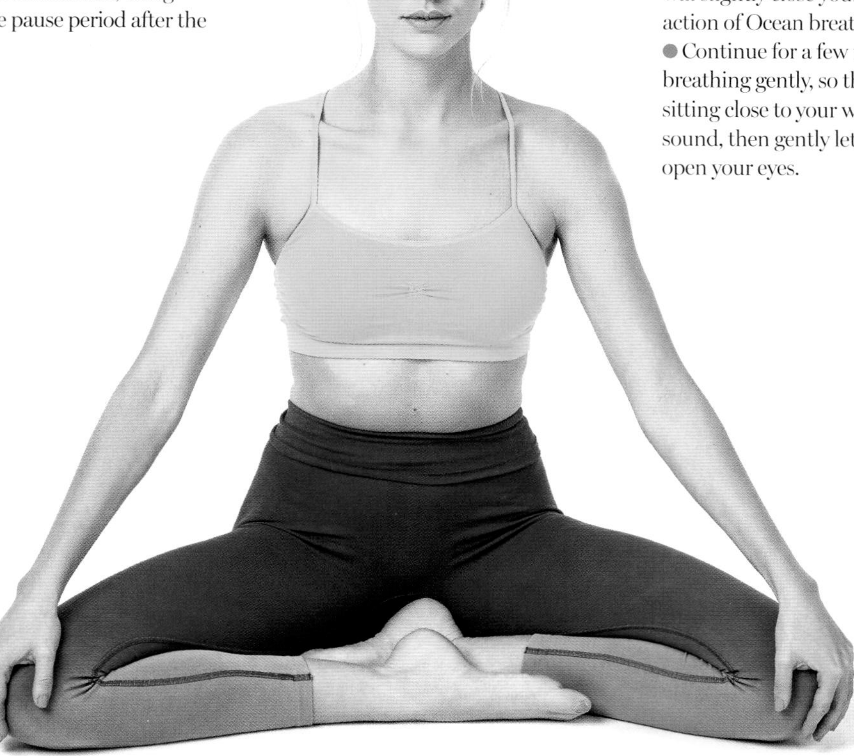

BELLOWS BREATH

KABALABHATI BREATHING

If you're feeling a bit sluggish or want to energise your whole body very quickly, a few rounds of Bellows breath will instantly refresh your mind and body, preparing you for any challenges ahead. Try it after a poor night's sleep or when you have a busy day in front of you.

- Sit in a comfortable position and close your eyes, breathing slowly and deeply into your belly until you feel calm and still, and ready to begin.
- Place your hands on your belly, inhale slowly, then draw your navel in and up as you quickly exhale through your nose. Pause, then repeat. Complete this sequence a few more times, while you become accustomed to the movement of your body on the exhalation. Then continue, but rather than consciously breathing in, see if you can allow inhalation to happen naturally. Once you feel comfortable with the technique, follow the sequence below.
- Repeat an inhalation/exhalation four to eight times, noticing how your belly moves in and out like a bellows beneath your hands. End with an out-breath. This is one cycle.
- Do another three or four cycles, gradually increasing the speed of your breath, so each exhalation lasts around one second. Take a few deep Ocean breaths (p98) after each cycle to rest your lungs and diaphragm.
- As you become more experienced, you can build up to 15–30 breaths per cycle.

* Do not practise Bellows breath if you are pregnant, menstruating or after eating.

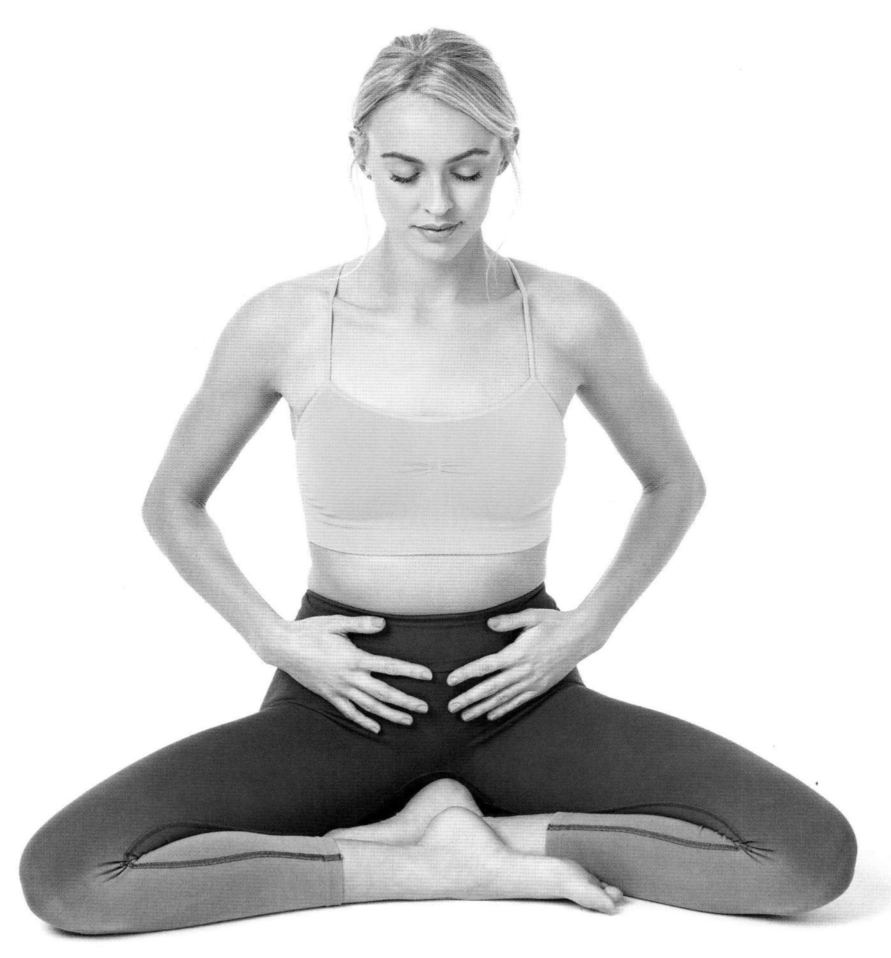

MORNING MEDITATION

There are many different ways to meditate, from counting your in- and out-breath to looking into the flame of a candle or resting your gaze on a religious symbol such as a Buddha. The technique you choose isn't as important as the quality of attention you bring to meditation. It's even possible to sit at your kitchen table, looking out at the sunlight glistening through the trees in your garden, and find a place of stillness.

All you need to meditate is to find a quiet place to practise, switch off your mobile phone and sit in a comfortable position – you can chose any of the meditation poses in this book, using a block or a bolster beneath your buttocks if your back is rounding. Or you may prefer to sit in a hard-backed chair – just make sure your feet are flat on the floor. To begin, gently close your eyes and spend a few moments arriving in your body. Your breath is the gateway to a meditative state, so always take time to settle into a relaxed breathing pattern before you start, taking slow deep breaths into your belly.

This meditation is ideal to use when you want to deepen your understanding about a situation, set some goals or intentions, or overcome any obstacles you may be facing. Use it when you have a challenging day ahead, at the beginning of a new a project, to help resolve a conflict with a friend or colleague, or simply when you're looking for more direction in your life.

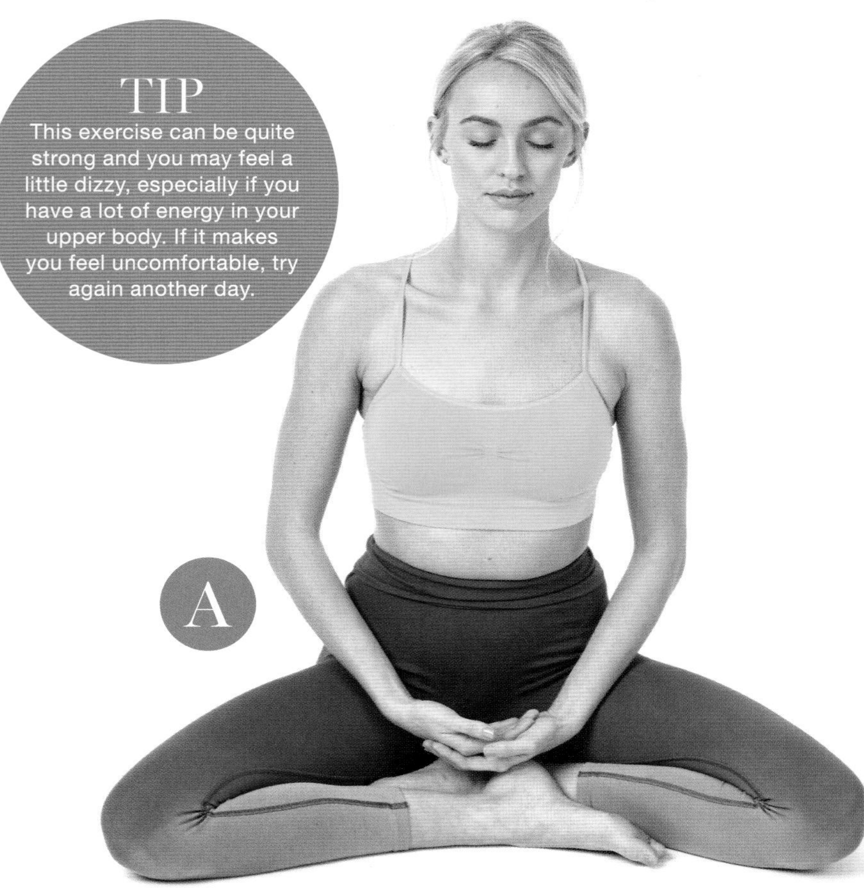

TIP

This exercise can be quite strong and you may feel a little dizzy, especially if you have a lot of energy in your upper body. If it makes you feel uncomfortable, try again another day.

FIND YOUR FOCUS

Being grounded is key to staying focused, so this meditation begins with an exercise to help you feel present in your body and be less susceptible to distractions. When you're not grounded, most of your energy is in your upper body – excessive energy in your head, for example, can express itself as an overactive mind, energy in your upper chest may show as a racing heart. The exercise in Part I helps move energy from your upper body to your lower body (legs and feet), to give you a more secure connection to your physical body and help you feel confident of your direction, both literally and figuratively. Allow 30-45 minutes for both parts of this meditation, or, if you have a regular yoga practice and already feel grounded, you can move straight onto Part II.

PART I

Stand with your feet hip-width apart and take your weight onto your right leg, bending your right knee slightly and keeping the ball of your left foot on the ground. Take your attention to the sole of your right foot then, in your mind's eye, slowly travel up your right leg to your right hip, noticing any sensations you feel. Perhaps you can sense heat, tingling or the pressure of the floor beneath your foot. Bring your awareness to the surface of your skin, then travel beneath your skin – can you sense your muscles and your bones?

Breathing freely, continue travelling from your hip – on your skin's surface or inside your body – to the area a few inches above your navel (solar plexus). Rest here for a few moments, imagining you have a nostril here and 'breathing in and out' from this place. When you feel ready, reverse the direction and travel back down your body to your hip, right foot and out

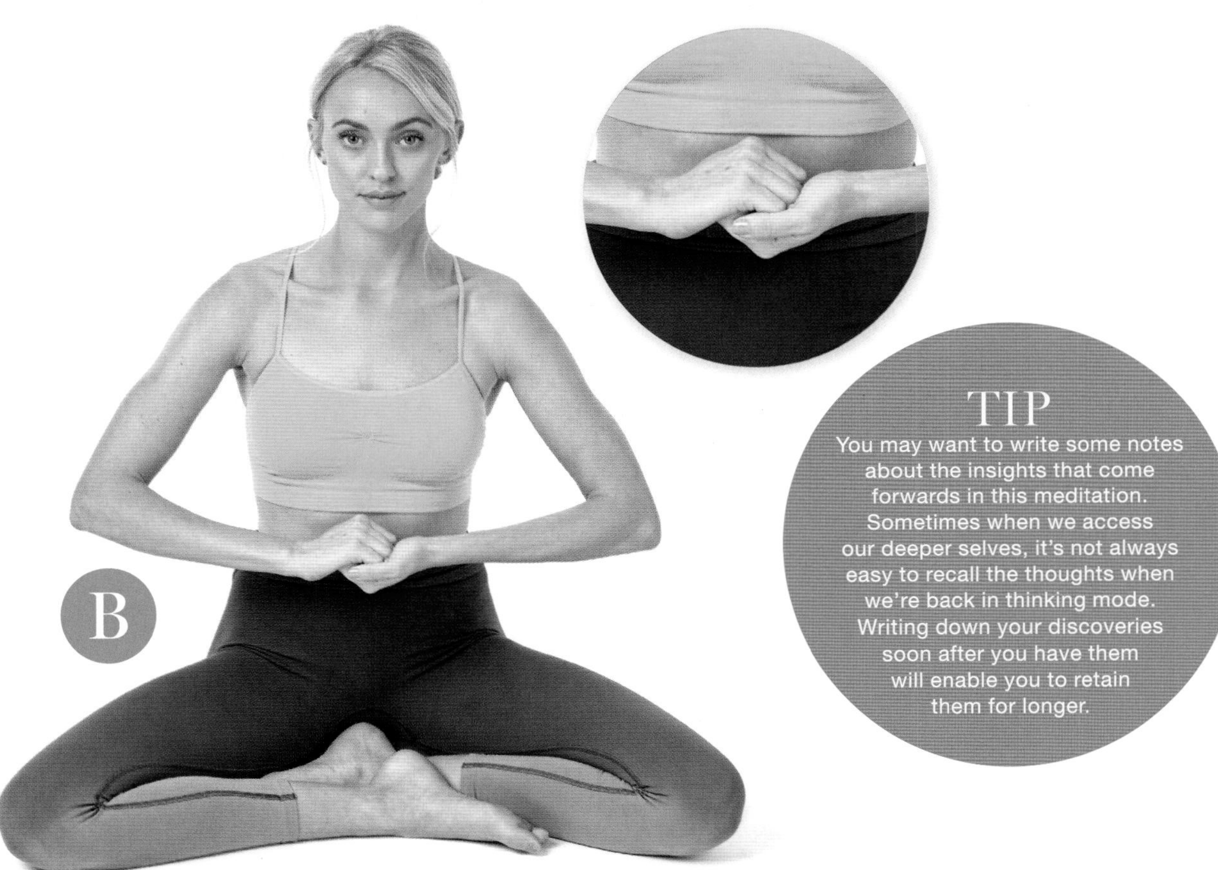

TIP

You may want to write some notes about the insights that come forwards in this meditation. Sometimes when we access our deeper selves, it's not always easy to recall the thoughts when we're back in thinking mode. Writing down your discoveries soon after you have them will enable you to retain them for longer.

through the sole of your foot into the floor. Pause for a moment or two, then repeat on your other leg.

In the final part of the exercise, bend both your knees, and simultaneously 'travel' up both legs to your solar plexus, then reverse the direction. When you've finished, rest for a moment in a comfortable seated posture before going on to your main meditation (A).

PART II

Take your attention to your sacrum and spend a few moments sensing the area. Then, when you feel settled, bring your attention to the front of your body, a couple of inches below your navel. Breathe deeply into this area for a couple of minutes and when you feel ready - you may feel your body becoming extra still or experience a heightened sense of awareness - reflect on the situation you've chosen, using the words Truth, Need and Priority as areas of focus. We've made some suggestions below to get you started, but allow yourself time to formulate questions that are meaningful for you, then let the answers naturally emerge from your deeper self into your conscious awareness.

Truth: What is the truth about this situation? What is real? If I wasn't feeling afraid/angry/hurt, what would I see?
Need: What do I most deeply need to do?
Priority: What matters most to me? What is my priority?

Finally, place your hands in the Ganesh mudra (B) – Ganesh is the Indian deity known as the remover of obstacles – and spend a few moments reflecting on any challenges you may face in your chosen situation. When you feel ready, release your hands, place them on your knees and rest your attention for a moment on the space between your eyebrows. Take a few final breaths, then gently release and softly open your eyes.

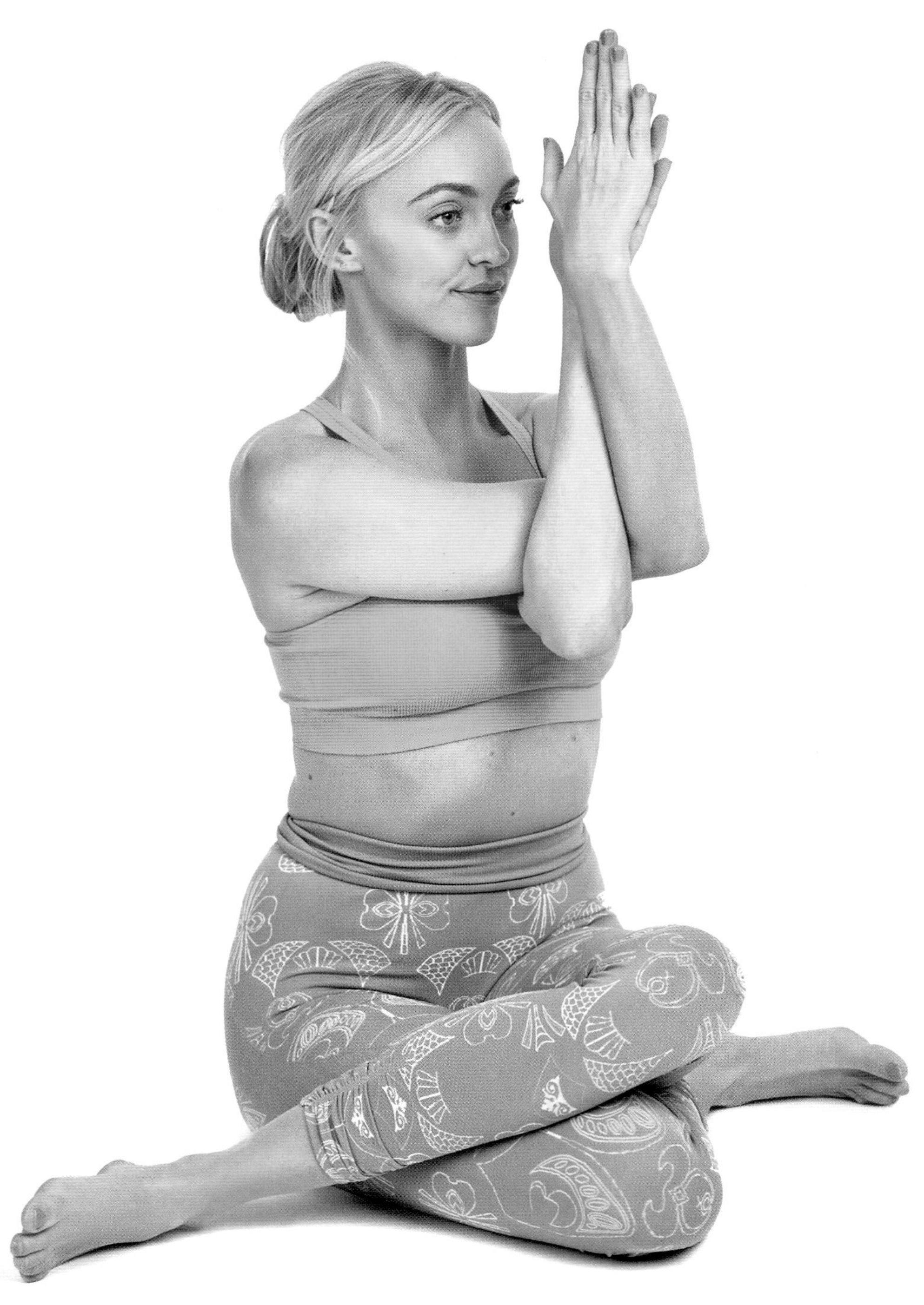

PM SEQUENCES

Ready for some chill time? This chapter begins with beautiful Qi gong moves to quieten your mood, then introduces you to five evening sequences to ease body and mind after a long day. You'll learn how to ease stress, switch off at will, improve your sleep and deeply relax. You can do the main sequences in 10 minutes, but for maximum benefit, set aside at least half an hour

QI GONG WARM-UP

Most of the PM yoga poses in this book are yin or restorative, so you don't need to warm up your body in the same way you would for a physically demanding practice. But it's a good idea to prepare yourself mentally. Letting go of a busy day or your unfinished 'to do' lists will enable you to get the most from your practice. The following warm-up is based on the Chinese healing system of Qi gong, and its slow, meditative moves are the ideal way to calm your thoughts, soothe your body and deepen your sensitivity to your moment to moment experience. Breathe gently throughout, inhaling through your nose and exhaling through your nose and mouth together. Move at a pace that feels right for you, and if you can do your practice barefoot, even better.

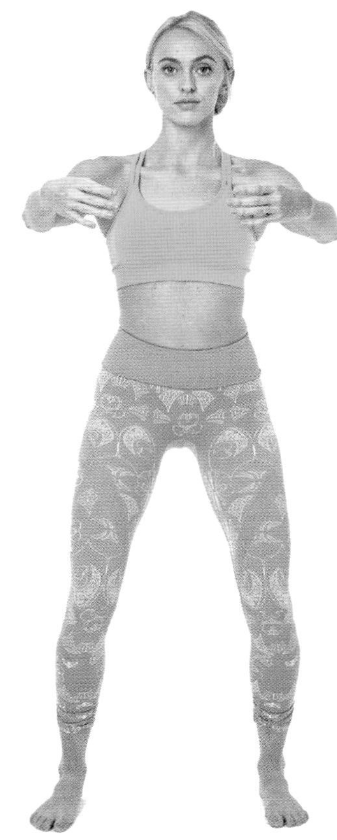

EMBRACE TREE

Stand with your feet parallel and shoulder-width apart, and softly bend your knees, letting your weight sink through your feet. Allow your tailbone to release towards the floor, to flatten your back, and let your arms hang limply by your sides. Lightly open your chest by releasing your shoulder blades down your spine and let the crown of your head float up to the ceiling. Bring your arms up to chest height, creating an open circle, with your palms facing you and fingers a few inches apart. Have a soft gaze, and rest the tip of your tongue behind the top of your front teeth. As you get used to the pose, as you inhale, imagine you're drawing energy up from the ground and through your feet into your body. Then as you exhale, imagine releasing tension downwards, from your upper body through your pelvis, legs and feet and into the ground. Rest in the pose for 30-60 seconds.

Benefits: Calming, grounding and aids focus.

PUSH HANDS

With your feet hip-distance apart, turn your left foot out 45 degrees and step forwards with your right leg, keeping your weight in your back leg. Bring your hands up to your chest, elbows bent and palms facing forwards (A), then on an exhale, transfer about 70 per cent of your weight onto your front foot as you simultaneously extend your arms forwards, still keeping your palms facing away from you (B). As you inhale, smoothly transfer your weight onto your back foot as you softly float your hands towards you, backs of your hands facing the ceiling, to the start position. Continue for a couple of minutes before repeating on the other side.

Benefits: Grounding, gently energising, strengthens your legs and back.

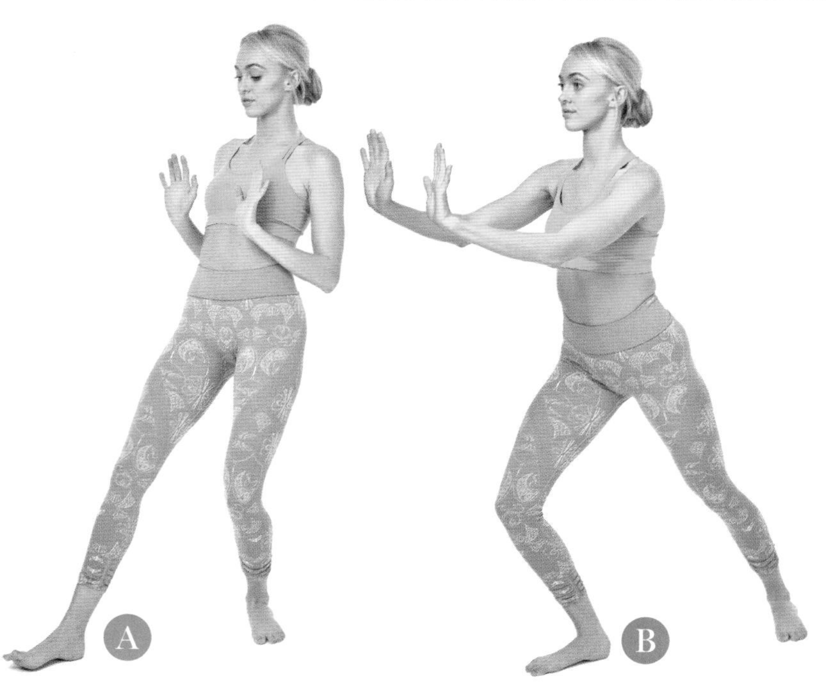

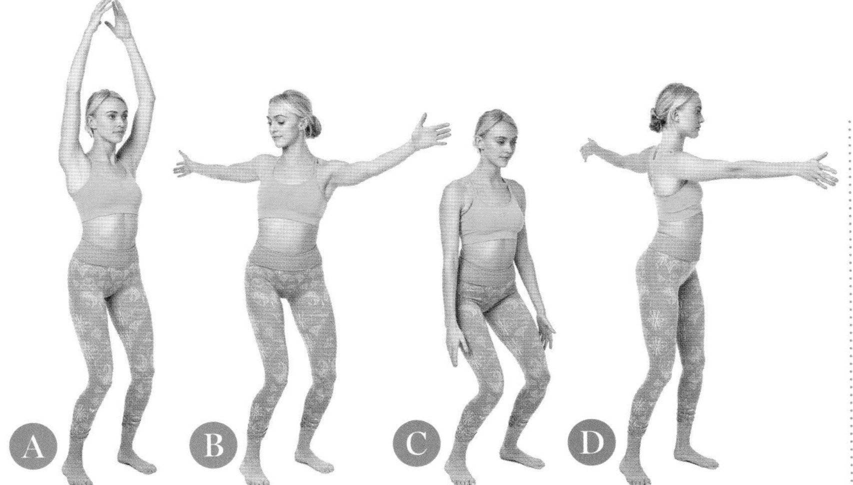

ARM CIRCLES

Stand with your feet hip-distance apart, knees softly bent and your arms over your head, hands lightly touching (A). Make large circles with your arms, simultaneously moving each arm in the opposite direction. Taking your left arm forwards and right arm back (B), bring both arms down and up. Your arms will meet at the bottom (C) and top of the circles (A). Do 10-20 circles and then switch direction, taking your left arm back and right arm forwards (D). Your torso naturally twists towards your back arm. It can take a few attempts to get used to this exercise, so start slowly and spend a few moments becoming accustomed to it. When you are comfortable, begin to increase the speed to the point where you naturally want to dip your knees as your hands reach the bottom of the circle. The breathing pattern is to exhale energetically as your arms move, pausing briefly as your hands reach overhead to take a quick breath in.

Benefits: Energises, warms your body, frees your shoulders.

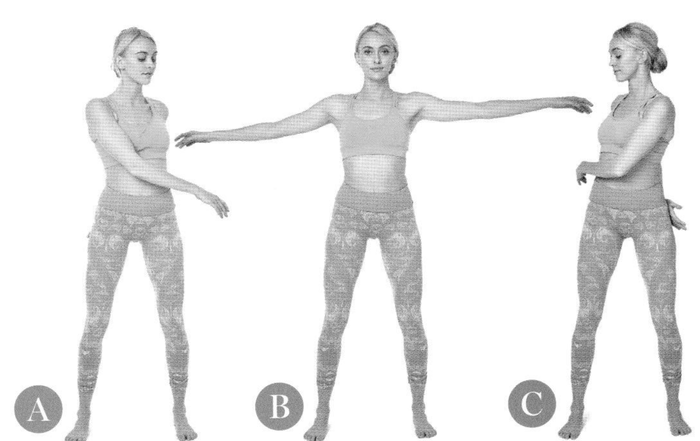

ARM SWINGS

With your feet shoulder-width, or wider, apart, begin to rotate your torso from right (A) to left (C), allowing your arms to swing around (B) as you do so. Starting slowly, let your arms completely relax, so they gently swing round your body like loose pieces of rope and your hands gently tap your sacrum and sides at the end of each rotation. Let your knees and pelvis be stable, facing the front, and gaze straight ahead to help prevent any dizziness. Breathe freely throughout and continue for one to two minutes.

Benefits: Loosens your spine, warms your body, tones your organs.

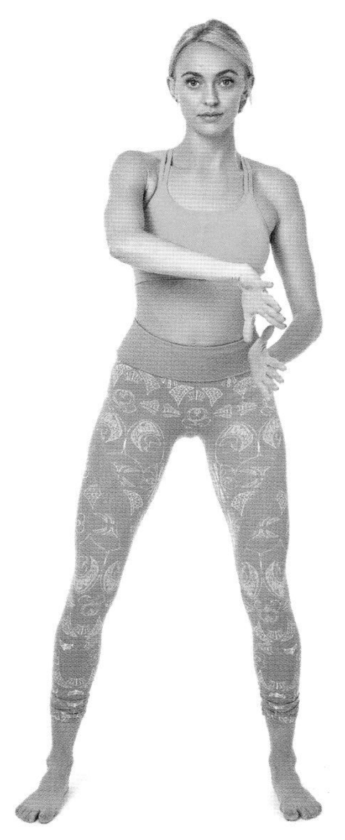

PUSHING THE WATER

With your feet shoulder-distance apart, take your hands in front of your left hip, your right hand stacked above your left and little finger uppermost and palms facing the centre. Keep your hands soft as you glide them across to your right hip, then switch hands so your left hand is over your right hand, again with your little finger uppermost and palms facing the centre. Continue gliding from side to side, moving in a slow fluid way, breathing freely and deeply. Gradually allow your torso to join in the movement, twisting slightly to the left as your hands move to the left and vice versa. You may find your left knee wants to bend as you twist to the left. If this is the case, simply allow it to follow the natural movement of your body.

Benefits: Strengthens your legs, loosens your hips.

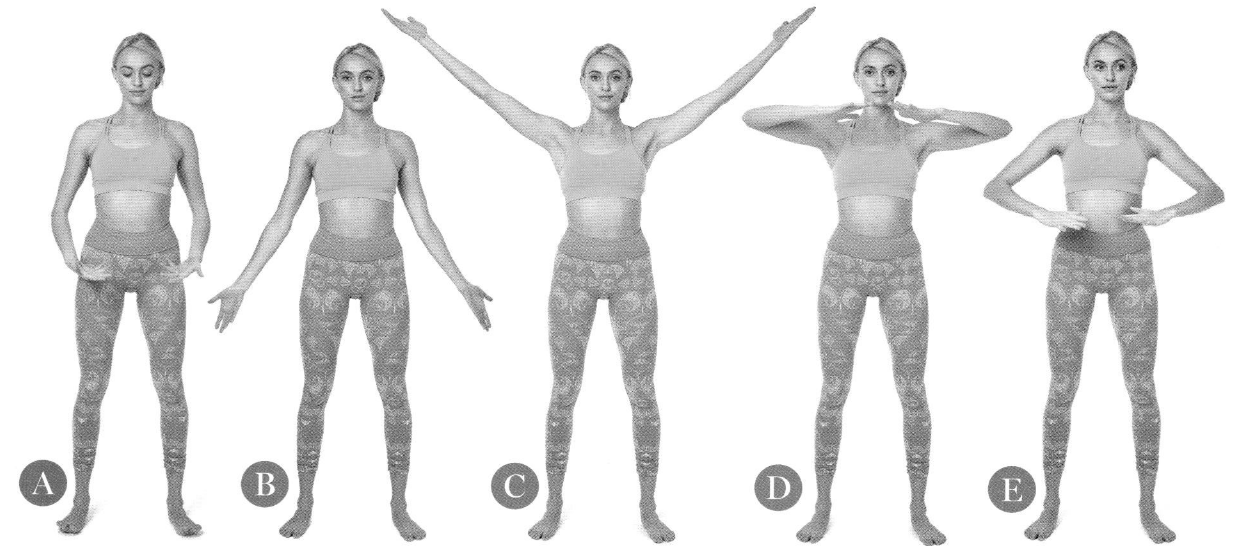

CLEARING

Begin with your feet hip-distance apart, knees soft, spine lengthening from your tailbone to your crown with your hands in front of you, palms facing upwards (A). Keep the back of your neck long and your shoulders releasing down your spine. With your eyes gently closed, inhale and trace your arms in a large circle out to the sides (B) and overhead. Keep your hands soft and palms facing upwards (C). When your hands are directly above your head, turn your wrists so your palms face downwards (D), and, as you exhale, spread your fingers and lightly press down as you bring your hands back to hip level (E). Imagine your hands are moving though water, creating a light resistance. At the bottom of the move, turn your wrists to face upwards again and repeat the circle, moving slowly and mindfully in time with your breath.
Benefits: Calms and stills your mind, grounds your energy.

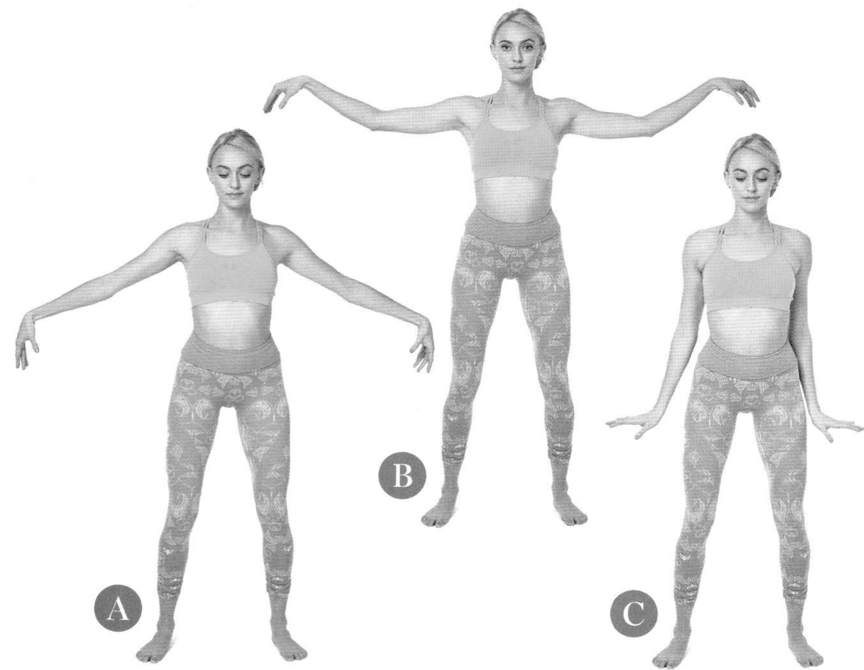

RAISE HANDS TO SIDE

A similar move to Raise hands (see opposite), this time your arms float up to the sides of your body. Begin in the same stance as for Raise hands, take a few breaths into your belly then on an inhale, slowly float your arms out to your sides, wrists soft and higher than your fingers (A). Continue until your arms reach shoulder height (B), then begin to release by exhaling, lowering your elbows, and letting your arms softly sink back to your hips, leading with your inner wrists (C). Raise your outer wrists as you repeat the upward motion once more. When you feel ready, introduce some movement in your legs by softly releasing your knees as your arms rise, grounding through your feet and straightening your legs as you lower your arms.
Benefits: Grounding, opens your side body, aids deeper breathing.

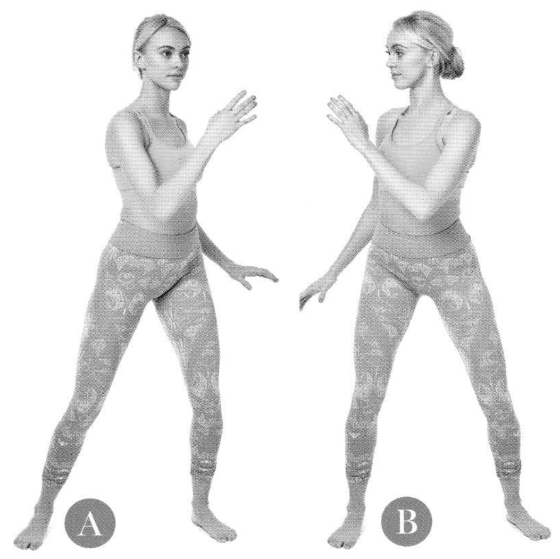

WAVE HANDS

Begin with your feet shoulder-distance apart, centre yourself, then bring your right arm in front of your chest, elbow down and palm facing your left. At the same time take your left hand towards your left hip, palm down, transferring your weight towards your left foot as you rotate your spine towards the left (A). Slowly swap the position of your hands, so your left hand is at chest height, your right by your right hip, and keeping your arms in place, rotate your torso to the right (B). Swap hands once more and twist to the left again. Breathing slowly and mindfully, continue alternating sides for a few more minutes.
Benefits: Releases tension in your spine, massages your inner organs.

RAISE HANDS

Stand with your feet shoulder-distance apart, knees slightly bent and crown lifting to the ceiling. Take a couple of breaths to centre yourself, then, as you inhale, float your arms up to chest height, leading with the back of your wrists. Let your elbows be slightly higher than your hands and your wrists soft, fingers relaxed (A). As you exhale, slowly lower your arms, leading with the inner wrists so your palms are directed away from you initially, facing the floor as your arms fully extend (B). Change your hand position, so the backs of the wrists lead. Repeat a few times more then begin to introduce slight movement in the legs, gently bending your knees as you raise your hands, straightening (but not locking) them as your hands lower.
Benefits: Deeply relaxing, stills your mind, slows your heart rate.

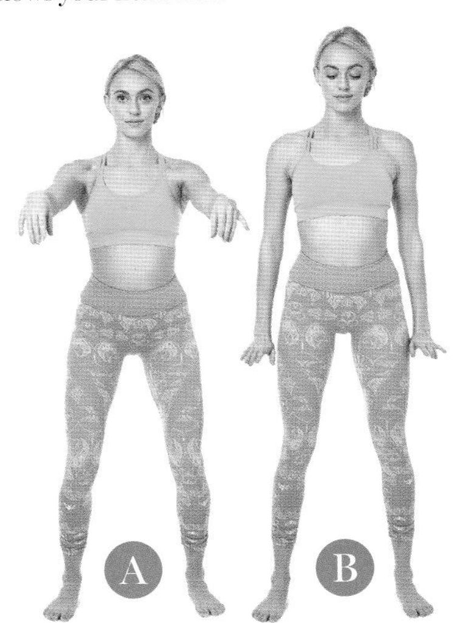

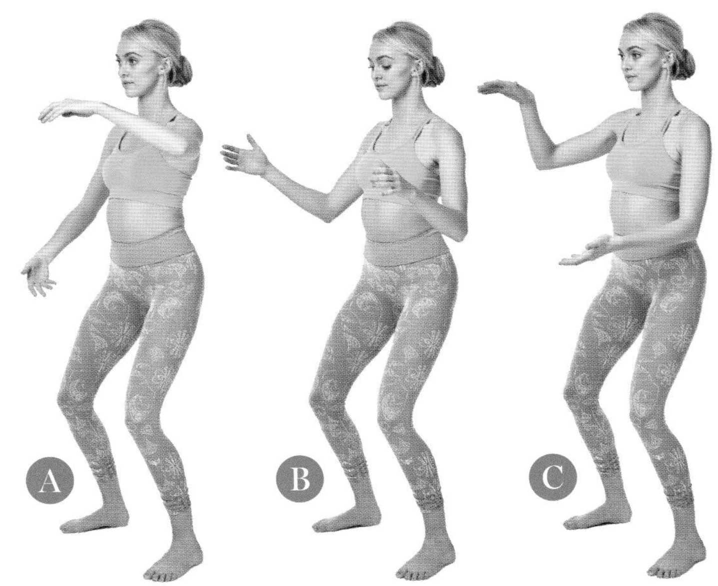

EMBRACE THE MOON

Spend a few moments centring yourself with your feet hip-distance apart, knees bent, tail bone tucked under and crown lifting, then bring your hands into Embrace tree (p104). Gently lower your right hand and cradle the space in front of you, as if you were holding a large ball. Slowly begin to circle your hands around the circumference of the 'ball' or 'moon' until your right hand is above your left (A), then reverse the movement, taking your hands back to your sides (B) and bringing your left hand uppermost (C). Breathing slowly and deeply, inhale and come to standing as you draw your hands out to the sides, exhale and lower as you bring them back to the mid-line. As you become familiar with the movements, gradually take your hand further out to the sides, expanding your body, breath and energy, before gathering everything in again and coming back to centre.
Benefits: Expands your chest, aids deeper breathing, increases your sensitivity to the movement of energy in and around your body.

MOON SALUTE I

Moon salutes make a beautiful alternative to Sun sequences when you are looking for a more gentle practice. As always, work with your breath, inhaling as you expand your torso, exhaling as you fold forwards. On your first round, aim to take three to five breaths in each pose, then follow the breathing pattern below for another two or three rounds. When you become familiar with the sequence, experiment by allowing the poses to merge into each other in one continuous flow.

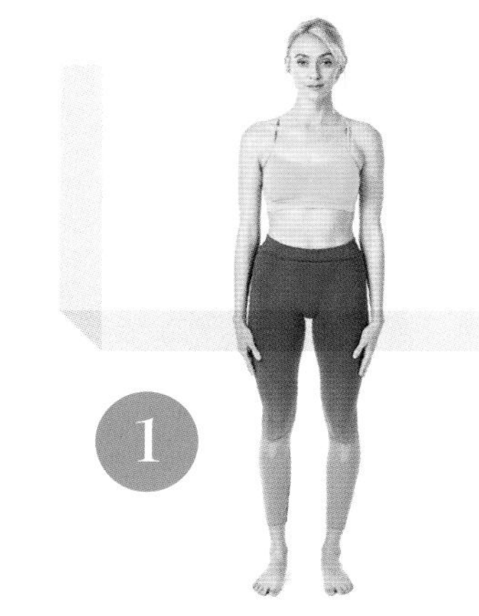

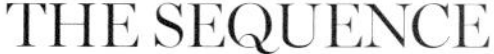

THE SEQUENCE

1 MOUNTAIN POSE
p44
Inhale, take your arms out to the side and overhead, and exhale into...

2 EXTENDED MOUNTAIN POSE WITH SIDE BEND
p44
Extend to the right, then inhale to the centre and exhale to the left. Inhale back up and step sideways with your left foot. Exhale into...

3 GODDESS
p37
Inhale. Turn your left foot out 90 degrees, and your right foot in slightly, and exhale into...

4 TRIANGLE
p55
Inhale, then exhale as you lower your right hand and turn both hips to the left, pivoting on your back foot, to come into...

5 PYRAMID
p47
Inhale, then exhale as you lower your right knee to the floor. Inhale into...

6 CRESCENT MOON
p29
Exhale and lower your hands to the floor and turn to your right into...

7 HALF SQUAT
p39
Inhale into prayer, then lower your hands and exhale into...

8 GARLAND
p36
Inhale into prayer, then lower your hands and exhale into...

9 HALF SQUAT
Inhale into prayer, then exhale as you lower your hands and turn to your right, lower your left knee and inhale into...

10 CRESCENT MOON
Exhale, lower your hands, then inhale and rise into...

11 PYRAMID
Exhale, then inhale, taking your left arm in a large arc into...

12 TRIANGLE
Exhale, then inhale to come up and exhale into...

13 GODDESS
Inhale as you step your feet together, exhale your hands into prayer. Inhale into...

14 EXTENDED MOUNTAIN POSE WITH SIDE BEND
Exhale to the left, inhale to the centre, exhale to the right, inhale back to centre, exhale into...

15 MOUNTAIN POSE
Pause, then repeat, leading with the opposite leg. This forms one round.

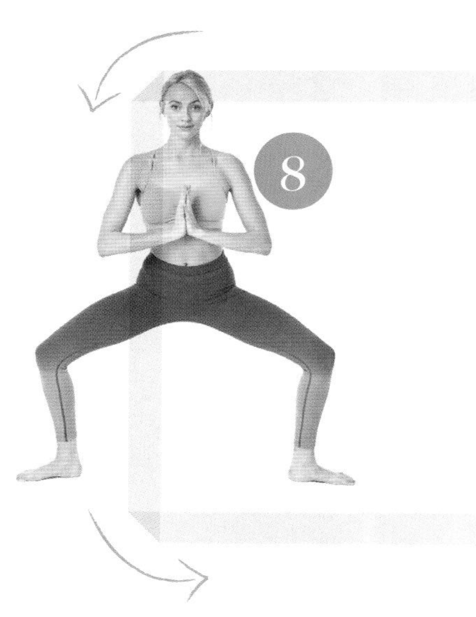

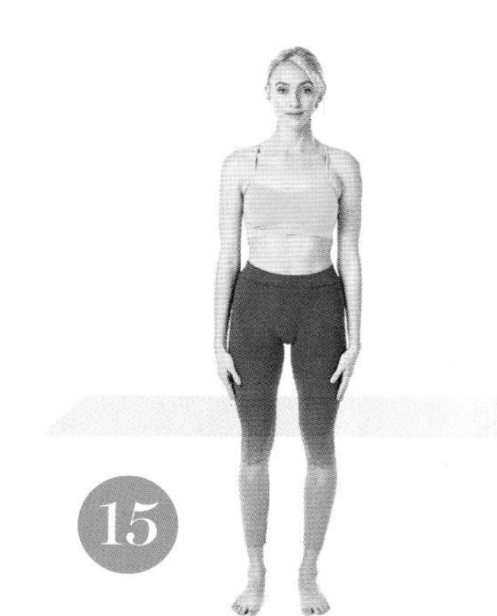

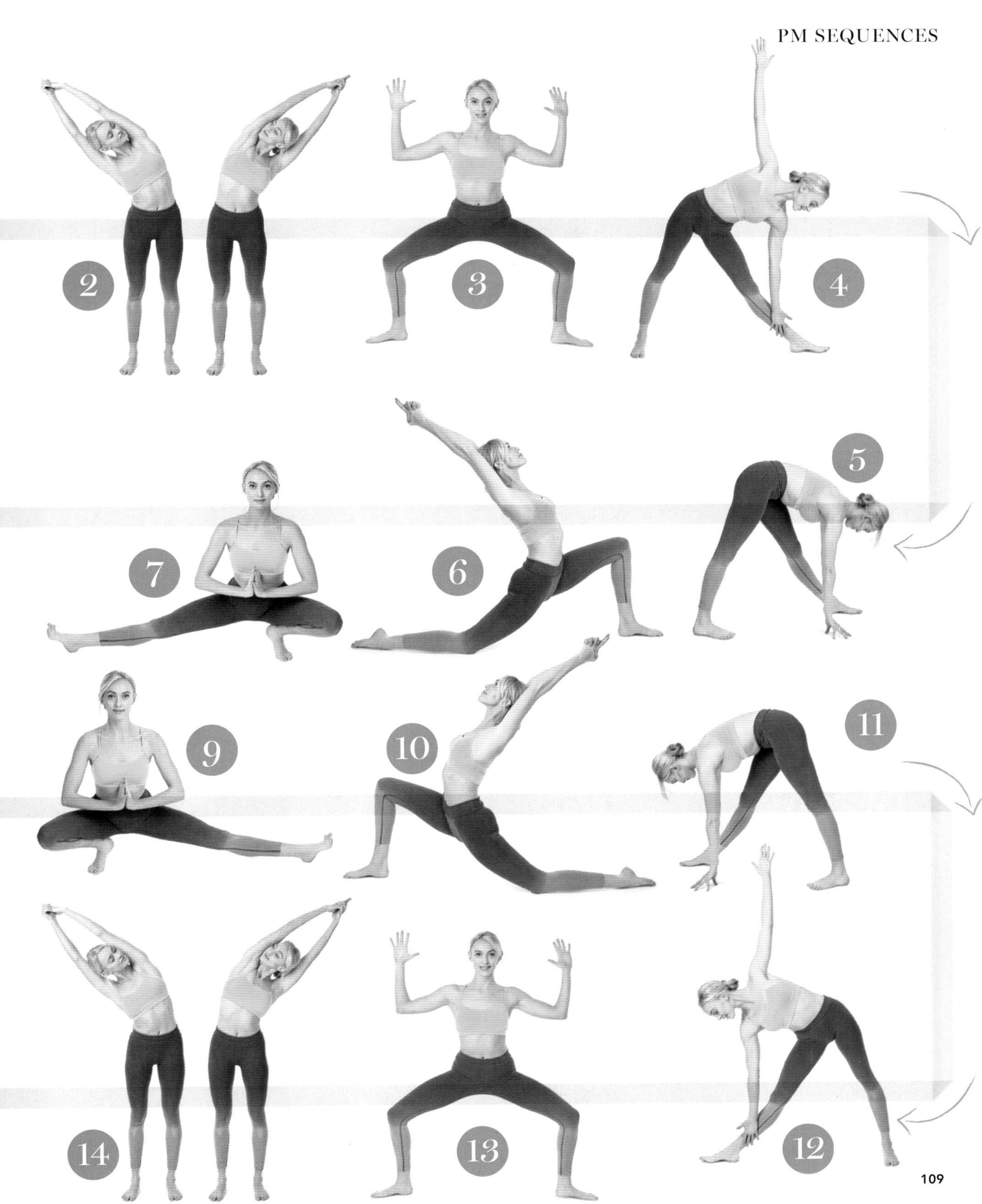
2
3
4
5
6
7
9
10
11
12
13
14

MOON SALUTE II

As you become more experienced, you won't need to mimic someone else's interpretation of a pose or sequence. Alignment points are guidelines only. In this Moon salute you'll practise freeform yoga, where you tune into your body and follow what it needs in the moment. Once you know the moves, let your body and mind surrender as you release and cascade from one to the next. Inhale as your heart expands, exhale as you fold forwards, or follow the suggestions below. If you want to repeat a move, stretch in a different way and notice how it affects your mind and body.

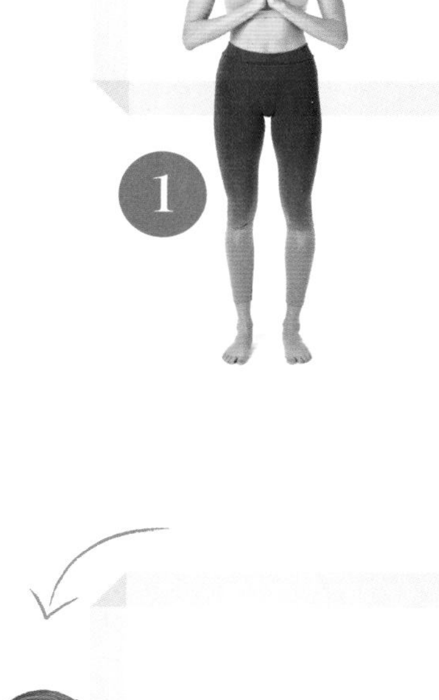

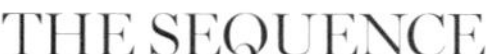

THE SEQUENCE

● 1 MOUNTAIN POSE p44
Stand in the pose, with your hands softly at your heart.

● 2 EXTENDED MOUNTAIN p44
Inhale, circle your hands out to the side and overhead. Inhale, root through your feet and lift through your chest into a backbend.

● 3 LUNAR STANDING FORWARD FOLD p52
Exhale as you fold from your hips. Keep your knees soft and let your chest drape over your thighs. Rest your hands on the mat, palms up. Inhale, step your left foot back then turn your front foot out 90 degrees and swivel onto the outside edge of your back foot.

● 4 NECTAR OF THE MOON I p45
Inhale to bring your right arm beside your ear. Ground through your left hand to lift and open your chest, keeping your legs active.

● 5 NECTAR OF THE MOON II p45
Exhale as you arc your right arm around towards your back foot.

Move between poses 4 and 5 three or four times, then pivot on your feet and walk your hands to your left so you face the long side of the mat into...

● 6-7 SPONTANEOUS FLOWING HALF SQUAT p39
Flow between your left and right feet a few times, gradually bending your knees to come into a deep squat. Finish by your left foot, place your hands either side of your foot and pivot to your left and step back into...

● 8 DOWNWARD DOG p30
Bring your feet hip-distance apart, lift your hips to the ceiling, ground your hands, rooting through the base of your thumbs and index fingers. Exhale into...

● 9 PUPPY DOG p83
Rest for a few breaths, then inhale as you come forwards to lower onto your stomach. Exhale. Inhale into...

● 10-12 SPONTANEOUS FLOWING COBRA p28
Rise up and down twice, letting your upper spine and shoulders move fluidly. Look to the right, tilting your shoulders and upper body to the right (10), then the left (11). Come into full Cobra (12). Lower to the floor on an exhale, rest, then inhale and root through your hands to lift into...

● 13 DOWNWARD DOG
Move freely as your body needs to for a few breaths, maybe slowly 'walking the dog' or circling your hips. Pause, then inhale and raise your left leg into...

● 14 DOWN DOG SPLITS
Exhale to lower your left leg as you bring it forwards into...

● 15 LUNAR STANDING FORWARD FOLD
Inhale and uncurl into...

● 16 EXTENDED MOUNTAIN
Root through your feet as you lift into your heart and crown. Extend your arms overhead, then lower, and pause, imagining you're being bathed in moonlight, then exhale into...

● 17 MOUNTAIN POSE
With your hands in prayer, tune into how you feel now. When you're ready, repeat the sequence on the other side.

9

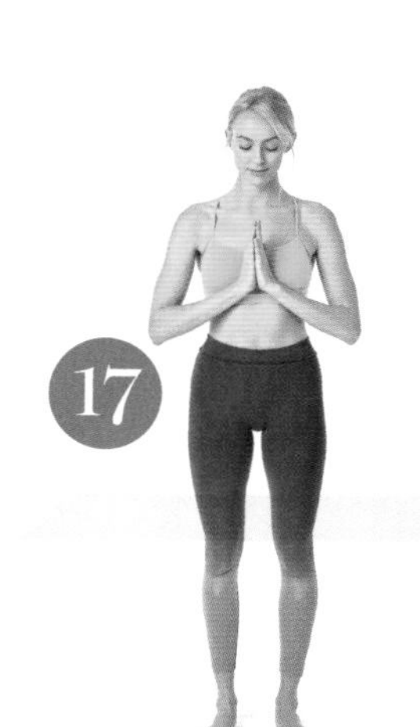

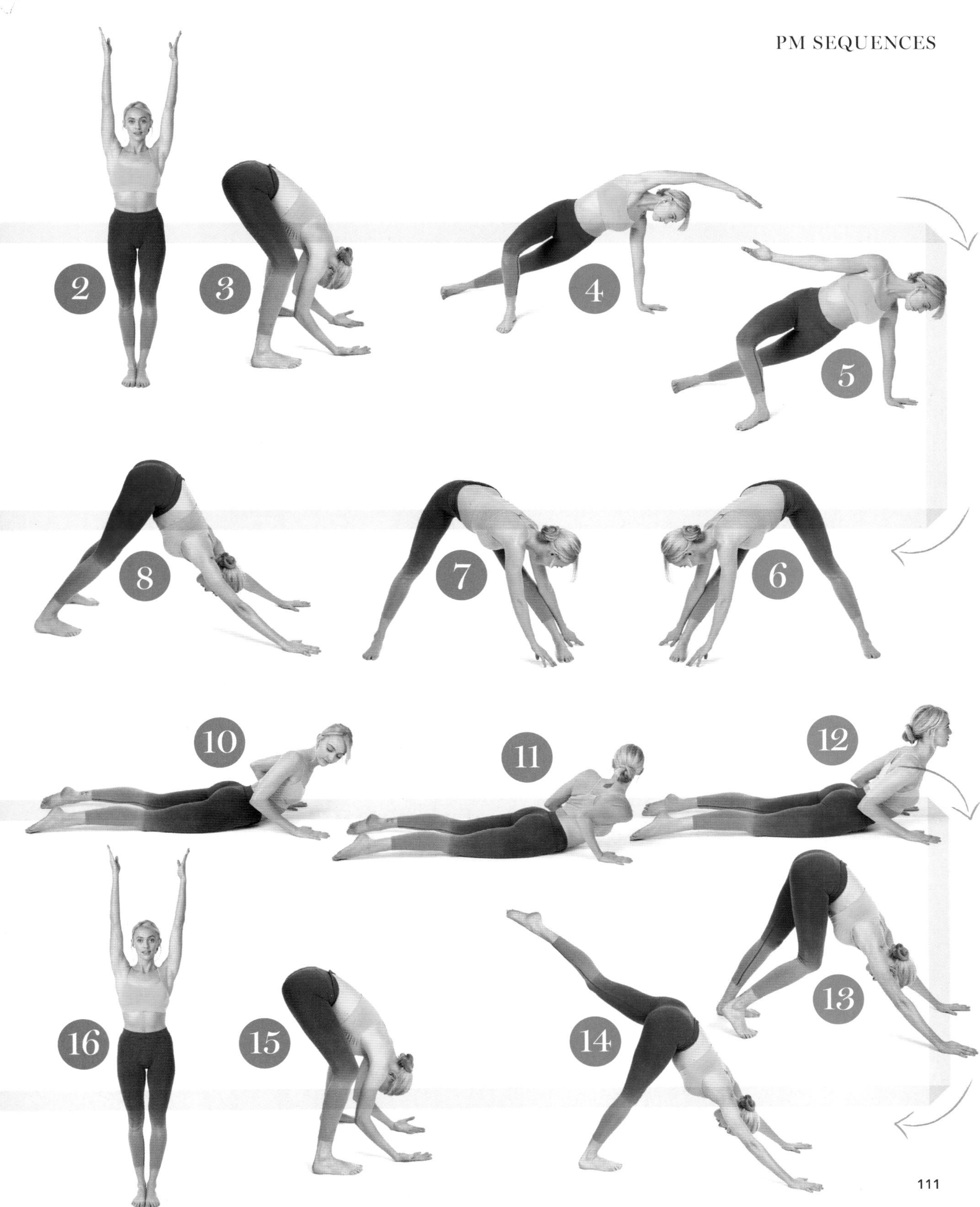
2
3
4
5
8
7
6
10
11
12
16
15
14
13

EVENING WIND DOWN

Whether you've had a long day hunched over a computer or have been running around after children, when the end of your working day arrives, a few restorative yoga poses can be hugely beneficial, easing tired legs, calming your mind and refreshing your system for the evening ahead. When you don't have a lot of time, spend three to five minutes in each of these poses and focus your attention on breathing deeply into your belly. If you feel you need a more restorative practice, you can rest for up to 15 minutes in each pose. When you have completed the sequence, if you feel you would benefit from some movement, do a couple of rounds of the flowing Moon salute I (p108).

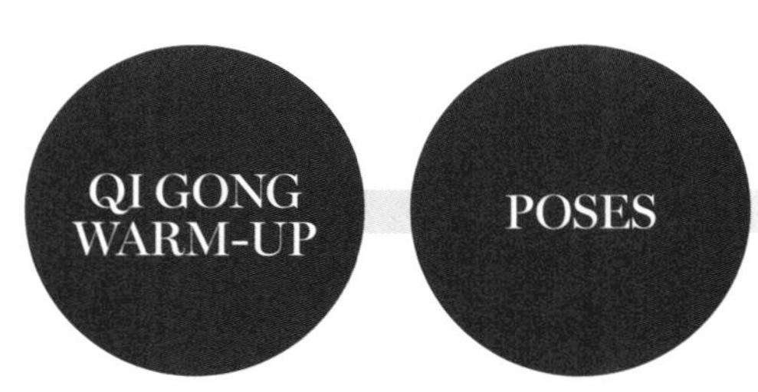

PROPS

Bolster
Blanket
Eye bag (optional)

QI GONG WARM-UP

A ARM SWINGS
p105

B ARM CIRCLES
p105

C RAISE HANDS
p107

D EMBRACE TREE
p104

E CLEARING
p106

POSES

1 LEGS UP THE WALL WITH BOLSTER
p65

2 BUTTERFLY
p62

3 RELAXATION POSE WITH BOLSTER UNDER CHEST
p67

4 RESTORATIVE TWIST
p70

5 RELAXATION POSE
p67

MOON SALUTATION II
p110

PRANAYAMA
Alternate nostril breathing
p123
Sit in any comfortable position, gently close your eyes and spend three or four minutes practising Alternate nostril breathing.

MEDITATION

Finish with the Simple meditation on golden light (p125).

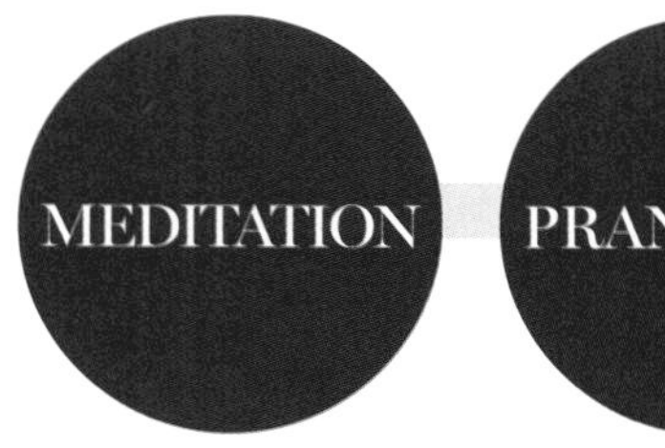

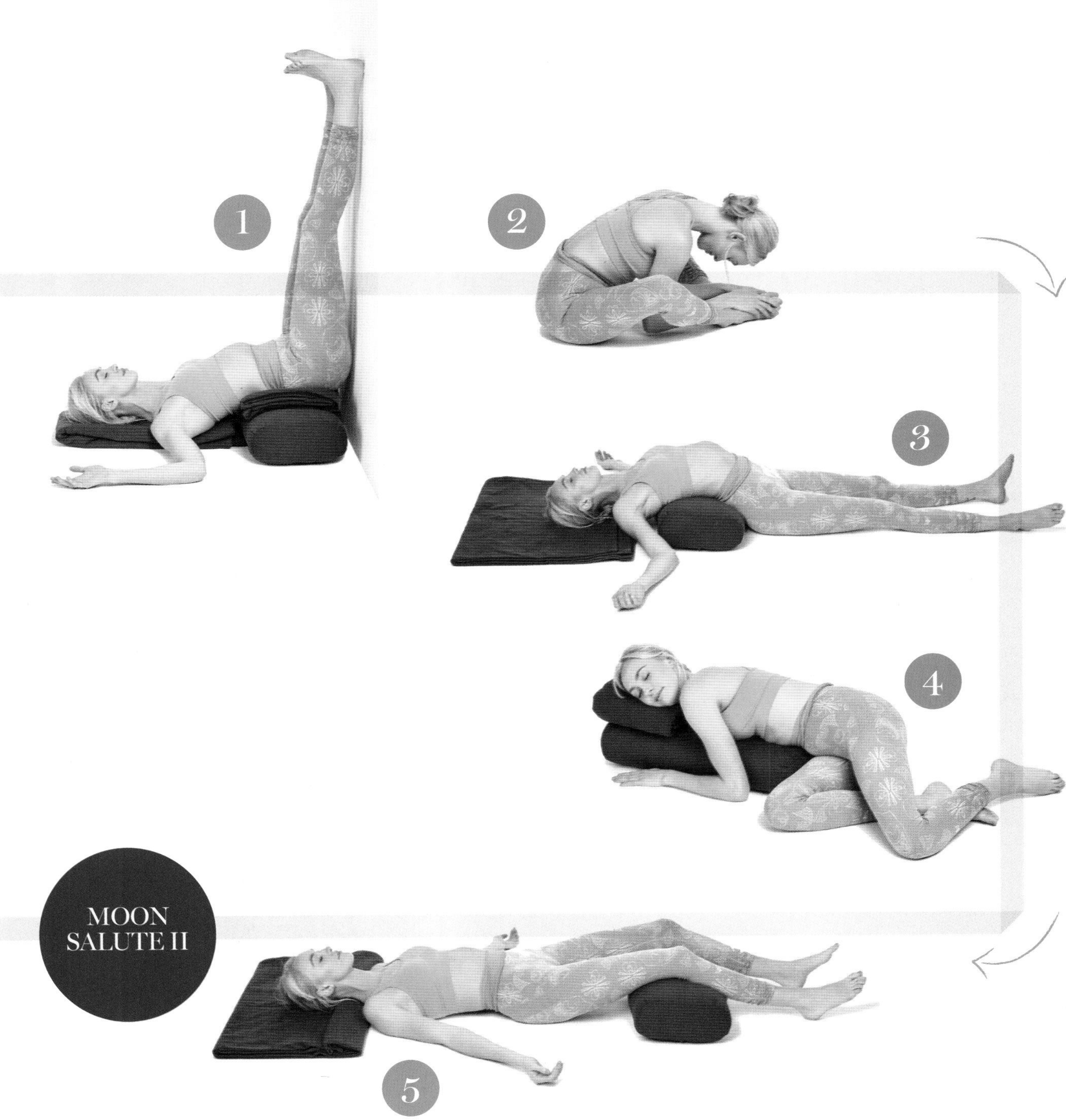
1
2
3
4
MOON
SALUTE II
5

DE-STRESS

When did you last take time out of your busy day to focus on rest and self-nourishment? All too often our hectic lifestyle means there's little space in the day for self-care. This sequence focuses on forward bends, which calm your nervous system and soothe your mind. The meditation is at the beginning of the practice, to help calm an overactive mind and prepare you for the sequences that follow. Breathe into your belly throughout, and if your mind wanders, gently return to your breath. Aim for three to five minutes (or longer) in each pose, but don't watch the clock, simply be aware of the feeling sensations in your body. As you do so, you'll begin to notice subtle changes occurring – a sense of sinking deeper into the posture as you release, a feeling of contraction or tension if you go too far. Trust your body – it will tell you when you're ready to move on to the next pose.

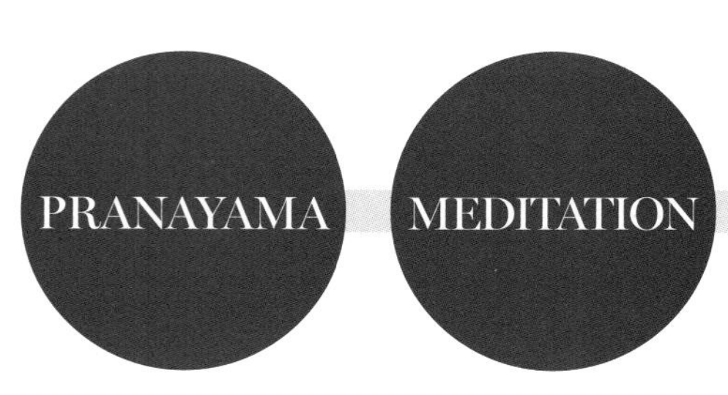

PROPS
Bolster and blanket
Block
Eye bag (optional)

PRANAYAMA
Full yogic breath in relaxation pose (p122)

MEDITATION
Simple meditation on golden light (p125)

QI GONG WARM-UP
A RAISE HANDS p107

B WAVE HANDS p107

C EMBRACE TREE p104

D EMBRACE THE MOON p107

E CLEARING p106

MOON SALUTATION II p110
Two to three rounds.

POSES
1 BUTTERFLY p62
Sit up in Easy pose (p33), place your hands on the floor behind you and gently bend backwards before coming into...

2 SLEEPING SWAN p73
Swing your back leg round to the front into...

3 HALF BUTTERFLY p62
Take your left leg out to the side. Then repeat poses 2-3 on the other side, lie on your back and do a couple of rounds of Windscreen wipers (p83) before coming into...

4 SNAIL p74
Lower onto your back with your knees bent, feet on the floor and gently raise your hips. Lower and come into...

5 HAPPY BABY p64

TO FINISH
6 RELAXATION WITH BOLSTER
Release your spine with Reclining twist (p48), then rest in Relaxation pose with a bolster beneath your knees (p67) and an eyebag over your eyes (optional).

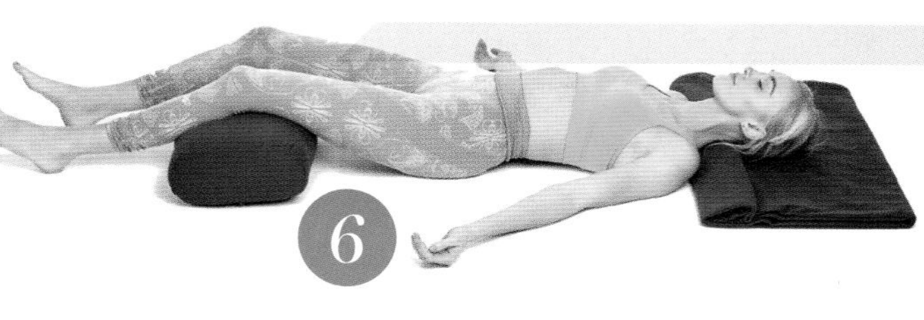

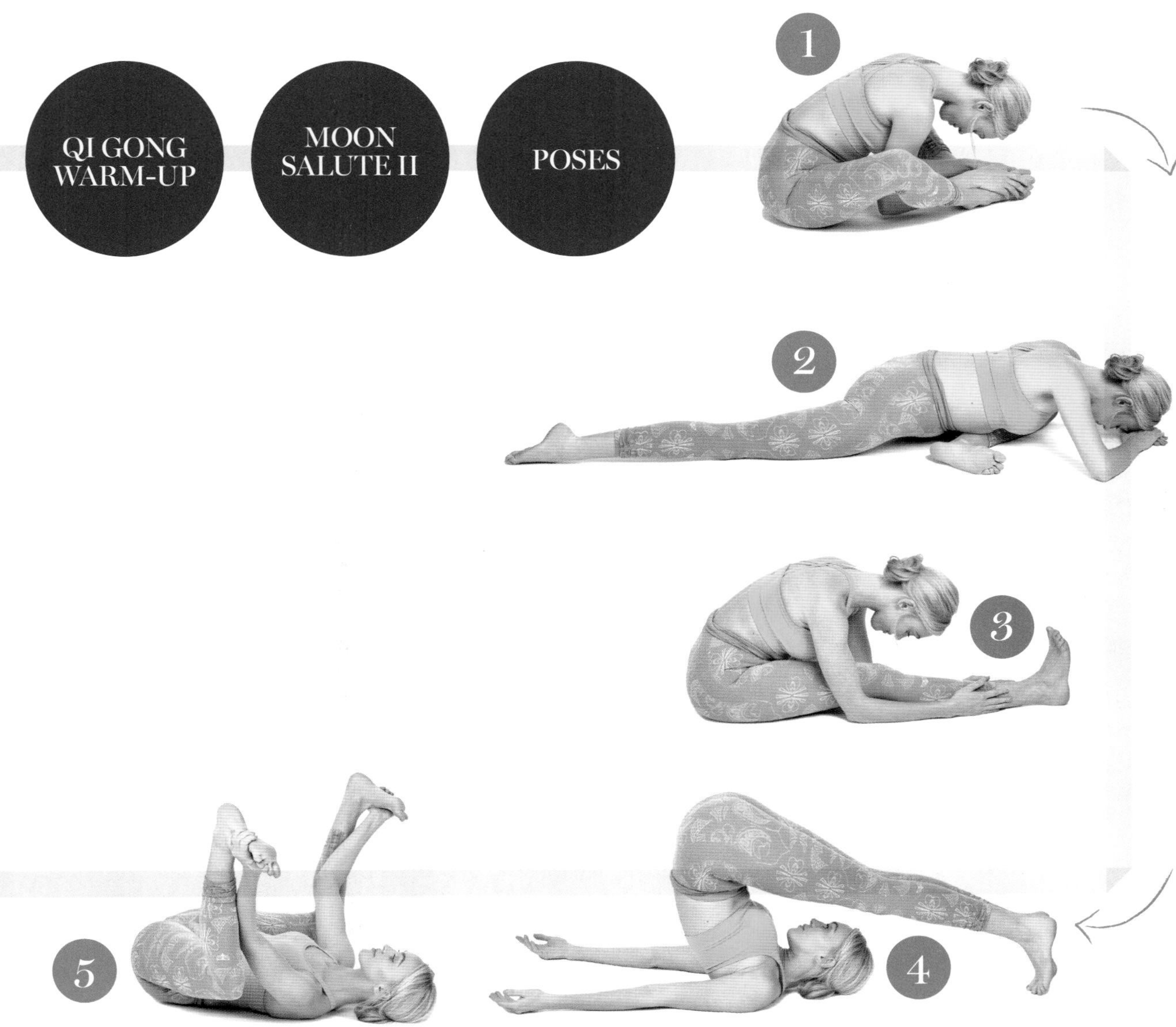
QI GONG WARM-UP
MOON SALUTE II
POSES
1
2
3
4
5

EVENING REFRESHER

This sequence is about balancing relaxation and stimulation. Begin slowly and gently with the Qi gong warm-up (p105) and Sun I/Moon I salute to let go of the day and attune to how your body and mind are feeling. Then, when you have a sense of how you feel now, tailor the main sequence according to your need. Work harder if you want to feel more invigorated (use Ujjayi breathing (p98), perhaps, or do each pose twice). Slow the pace if you want to feel gently refreshed.

The Sun salute opens the front and back of your torso, while the Moon salute works the sides. The twists compress and release tension from your spine, allowing fresh blood and oxygen to flood the area, while the inversion (Snail) invigorates the brain. The backbends open the chest area and energise your system. You can adjust the depth of your backbend according to how stimulating you want the pose to be, for example, chose Seal over Sphinx if you have an active evening planned and want to feel more energised.

QI GONG WARM-UP

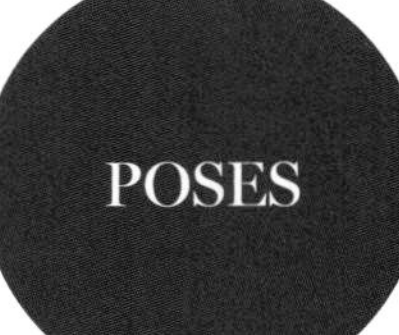

PROPS

Block or blanket

QI GONG WARM-UP

A ARM SWINGS
p105

B ARM CIRCLES
p105

C EMBRACE TREE
p104

D PUSH HANDS
p104

E EMBRACE THE MOON
p107

SUN SALUTE I
p84
One to two rounds.

MOON SALUTE I
p108
One to two rounds.

POSES

1 SHOELACE p72
Do the pose on both sides.

2 SPHINX OR SEAL p75

3 TWISTED DRAGON
p76
Do the pose on both sides.

4 SADDLE OR HALF SADDLE
p71
If doing half saddle, do the pose on both sides.

5 SNAIL p74

PRANAYAMA
A few rounds of Ujjayi breathing (p98) will give you a quiet, calm strength or, if you have a busy evening planned, Bellows breath (p99) will leave you energised and ready to go.

MEDITATION

Do Simple meditation on golden light (p125).

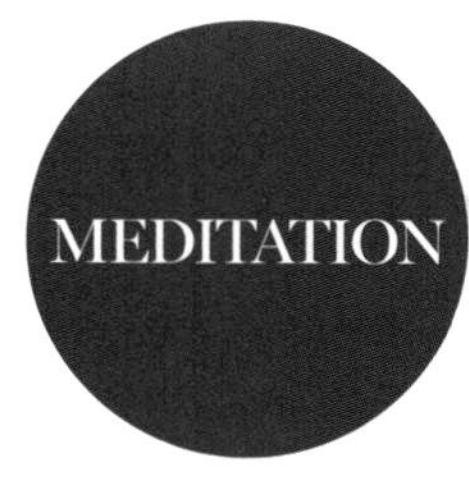

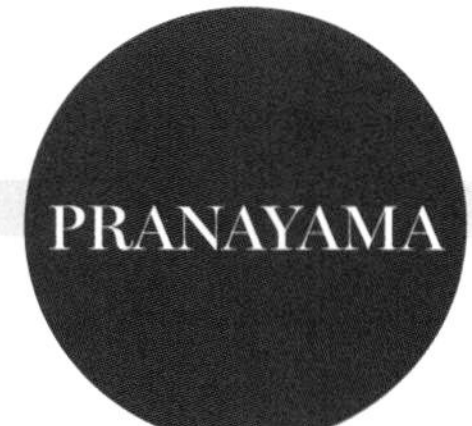

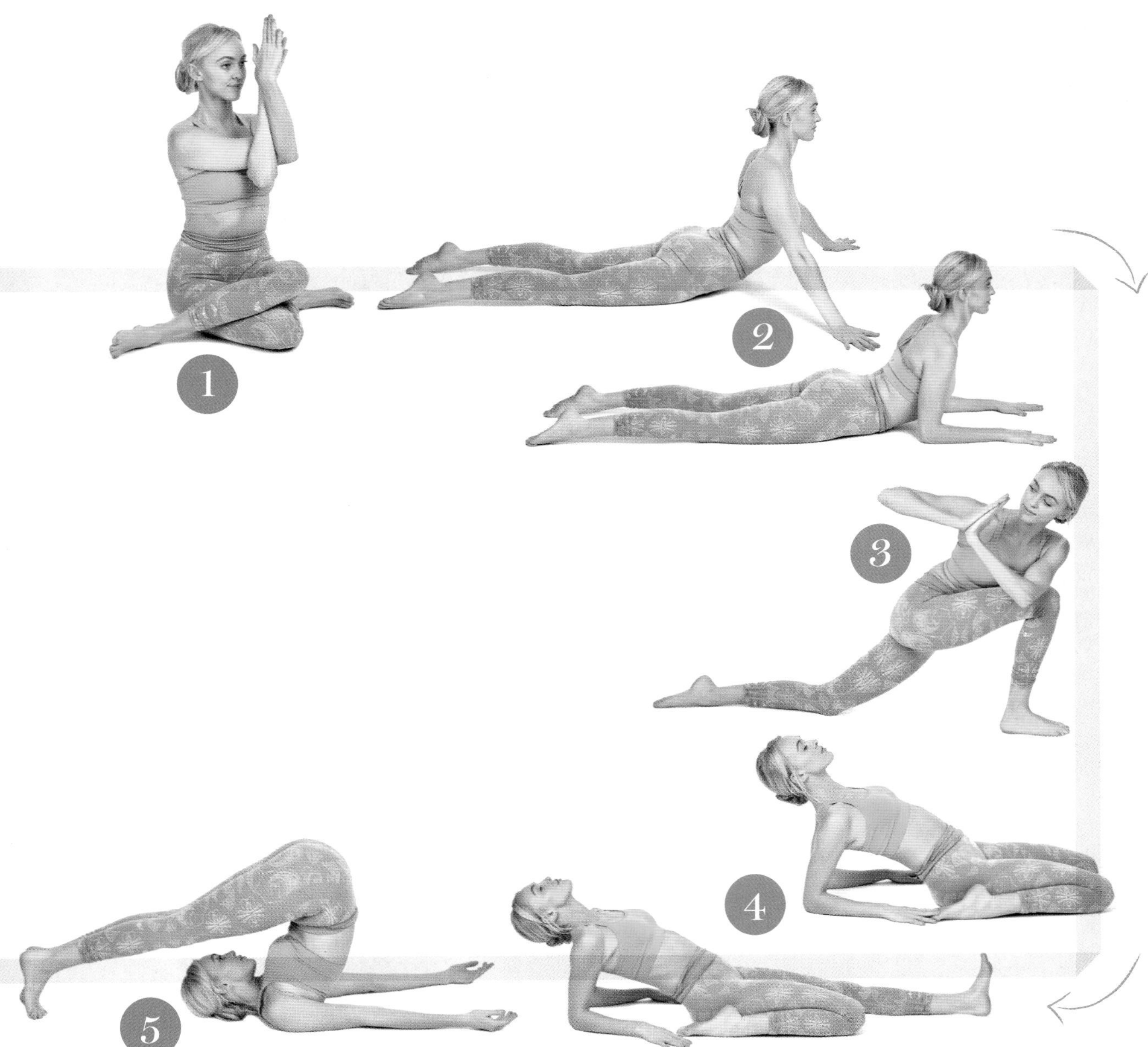
1
2
3
4
5

SWEET DREAMS

Anxiety, an overactive mind or eating too late in the evening can all interfere with your ability to fall asleep, but these calming poses will soon have you drifting off. Move slowly and sensitively, particularly in the transitions between poses, so you don't disturb the sense of relaxation you've built up. And, if possible, do the Evening wind down sequence when you arrive home after work, that way you won't carry the tension of the day through to bedtime. To feel even more relaxed, spray the top of your eye bag with lavender pillow mist and use it in Relaxation pose and for Yoga nidra – the essential oil has been proven to calm the activity of the brain.

Ideally, spend three to five minutes in each pose - or longer if you have time. When your insomnia is particularly challenging, or if it's 3am and you're feeling exhausted from lack of sleep, try doing the main poses in bed using your pillows in place of a bolster, that way you can simply drop off when your mind and body are sufficiently relaxed. It's quite common to fall asleep during Yoga nidra, so if you're not already there, get into bed before you begin the closing meditation.

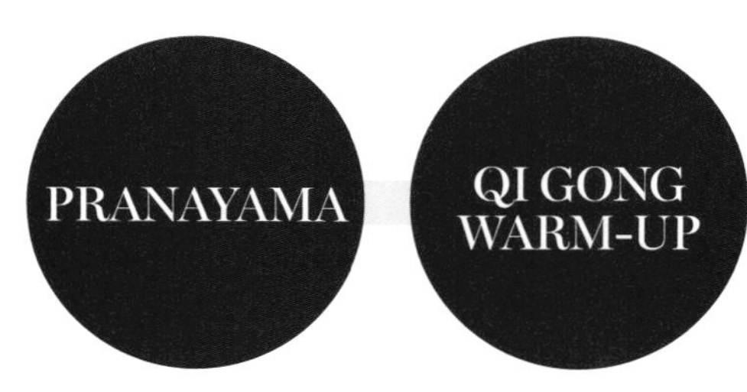

PROPS

Bolster (or pillows if in bed)
Blankets
Strap
Eye bag
Lavender pillow mist

● **PRANAYAMA**
Full yogic breath (p122) in relaxation pose.

QI GONG WARM-UP

● **A RAISE HANDS**
p107

● **B EMBRACE THE MOON**
p107

● **C RAISE HANDS TO SIDE**
p106

● **D PUSHING THE WATER**
p105

● **E CLEARING**
p106

● **MOON SALUTE II**
p110

POSES

● **1 RESTORATIVE CHILD'S POSE**
p69

● **2 RESTORATIVE TWIST**
p70
Do the pose on both sides.

● **3 RESTORATIVE BUTTERFLY**
p68

● **4 CAT PULLING ITS TAIL**
p63
Do the pose on both sides.

● **5 RELAXATION POSE**
p67
Place a bolster or pillows beneath your knees.

MEDITATION

Do Yoga nidra (p124).

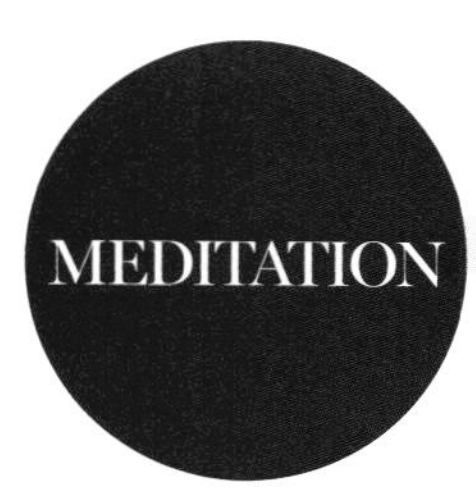

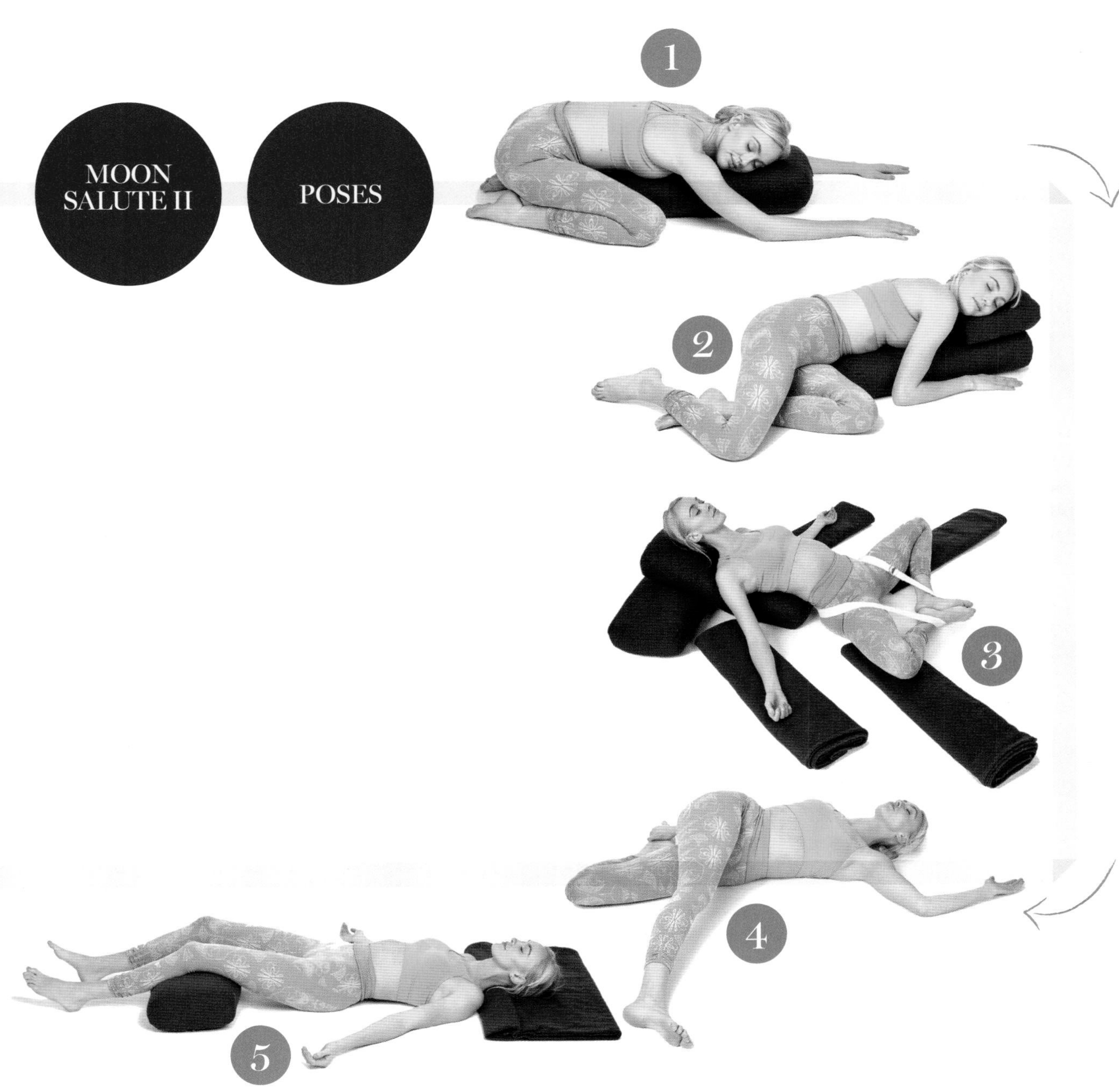
MOON
SALUTE II
POSES
1
2
3
4
5

DEEPLY RELAX

We very rarely relax deeply, but when we do, it has an immensely healing effect on both our mind and body. Being relaxed can give you a quiet confidence that has great strength, your immune system will function more effectively and your problems may seem smaller. Our systems are so often overloaded with stimulation that it takes time for your body to become calm, so in this sequence, to reap the most benefits, aim to spend 10 to 15 minutes in each posture. Breathe into your lower belly, and make your exhalation longer than your inhalation to activate the relaxation response of your nervous system. If you've come from a particularly busy day, burning a scented candle, some lavender essential oil or playing your favourite calming piece of music will help you transition into a quiet space.

When you've completed the main sequence, check in with your body/mind and, if it feels right, you might like to explore how it feels to move from a place of deep relaxation. So often in yoga, as in life, we force ourselves to go against our natural rhythm in order to achieve a goal. Today, use Moon salute II as an opportunity to practise moving without creating a disturbance to the sense of relaxation you've built up, and notice how different the experience feels.

QI GONG WARM-UP

POSES

PROPS

Bolster
Blocks
Blankets
Strap
Eye bag

QI GONG WARM-UP

A EMBRACE TREE
p104

B RAISE HANDS
p107

C WAVE HANDS
p107

D PUSH HANDS
p104

E CLEARING
p106

POSES

1 RESTORATIVE BUTTERFLY
p68

2 MOUNTAIN BROOK
p66

3 WIDE-LEG SEATED FORWARD FOLD
p77

4 RESTORATIVE TWIST
p70
Do the pose on both sides.

5 RELAXATION POSE
p67

MOON SALUTE II (OPTIONAL)
p110
When you've finished the Moon salute, pause for a moment in Mountain pose (p44), then finish with three rounds of Clearing (p106).

MEDITATION

Come into any comfortable position and breathe softly through your nose for a few moments, then begin the Simple meditation with golden light (p125).

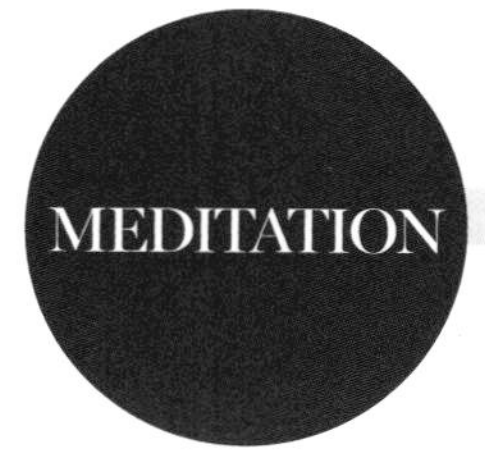

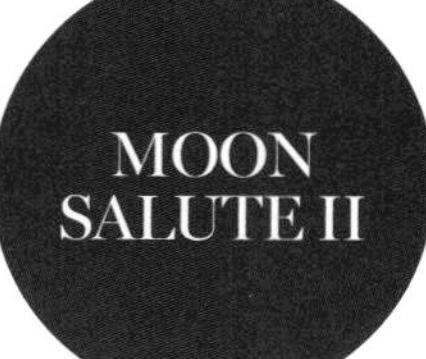

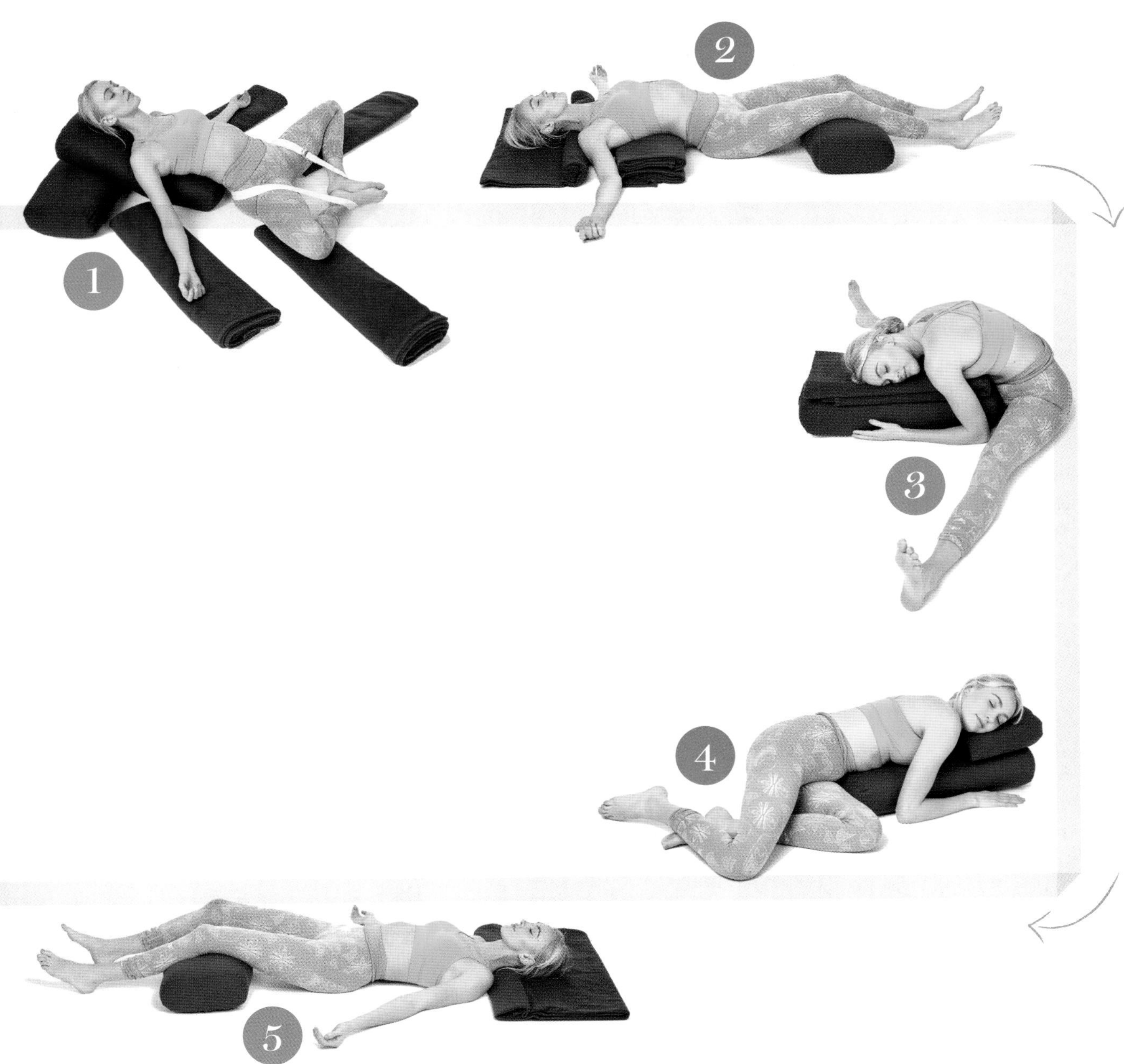
1
2
3
4
5

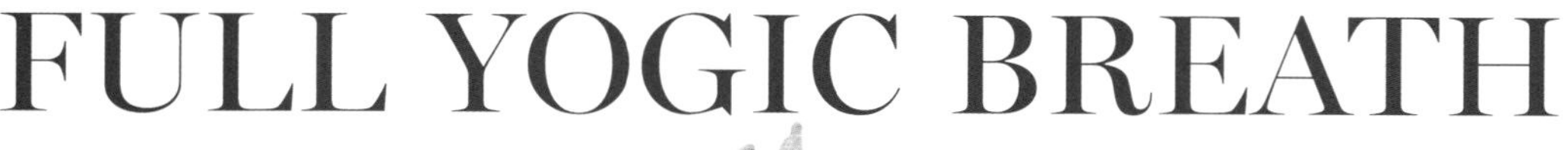

FULL YOGIC BREATH

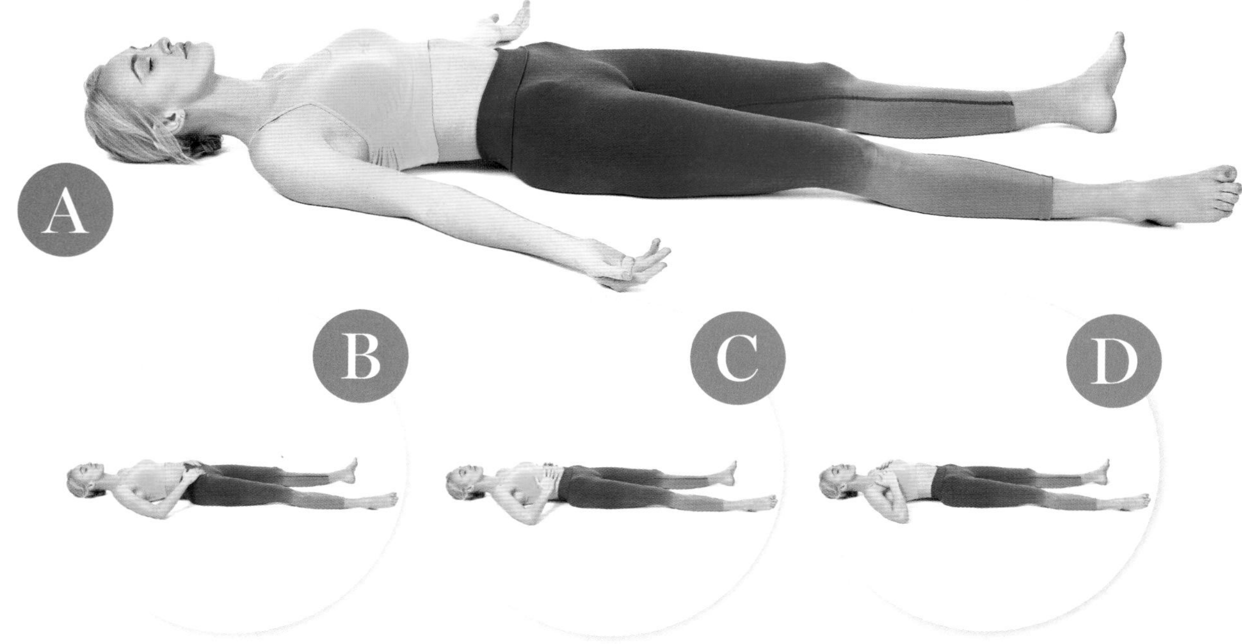

We rarely use the full capacity of our lungs, but breathing fully and deeply has a wealth of benefits, from calming the mind, and increasing focus and concentration to helping you make better decisions. In your evening yoga practice, breathing well will be deeply relaxing, and allow you to tune into your moment by moment experience, so you can enjoy maximum benefits of the sequences. As you are learning the full yogic breath (below), allow 15 to 20 minutes for the practice. Once you become familiar with the technique, you'll be able to drop into full yogic breathing at will.

- Lie on your mat in Relaxation pose, gently close your eyes and spend a few moments allowing your breath to settle and your mind to become calmer (A).
- Take a deep breath in through your nose, then exhale through your mouth, letting go of any tension on your out-breath. Do this a couple of times, releasing any thoughts. It's important that you're comfortable here, so make any adjustments, then let your breath settle and your heartbeat quieten.
- Focus on your breath and become aware of your natural breathing pattern. Are you breathing quickly or slowly? Are you taking a full in-breath and completely emptying your lungs when you breathe out? Observe how you are breathing in this moment.
- Become aware of any movements in your body as you breathe. Can you feel your chest expanding or your belly rising? Take your attention to the back of your body so you can sense it pressing slightly into the mat as you inhale. Tune in to your body's micro-movements as you breathe in and out.
- Place your hands on your lower belly, beneath your navel, with your fingertips touching and the heels of your hands resting on your hips (B). Allow your belly to soften and become aware of it rising as you inhale, and gently falling as you exhale.
- Now, slide your hands to your side ribs, thumbs beneath your back, fingers wrapped round your front ribs (C). As you breathe, can you feel any movement beneath your hands? If you're finding it hard to sense anything, gently draw your abdomen towards your spine. Continue for a few breaths, following your natural rhythm, and tuning in to the movement of your ribs as they respond to the action of your diaphragm, the main breathing muscle.
- Finally, slide your hands to your upper chest (D). Can you sense any micro movements here? To practise a full yogic breath, begin to direct where your breath travels to, first filling your abdomen, then your ribs and finally your upper chest, as if you were filling a vase with water – first the base, then the middle and lastly the neck.
- As you exhale, empty from your chest, then your ribs and lastly your belly.
- Like the vase, your diaphragm and lungs are three-dimensional, so allow your breath to travel to the back and sides of your body as well as the front. Continue in your own rhythm for a few breaths, then gently let your breathing return to normal.

ALTERNATE NOSTRIL BREATHING

NADI SHODHANA

Alternate nostril breathing is traditionally used to balance the left and right sides of the body. You can use this practice whenever you want to ease anxiety or still your mind.

- Choose a comfortable position to sit on your mat and rest your hands on your knees, using a block beneath your sitting bones if your back is rounding. Spend a few moments letting your breath settle, taking a few deep breaths into your belly and feeling your body relaxing more and more on each exhale.
- When you feel ready to begin, bring your right hand to your nose, rest the tip of your thumb on the fleshy part of your right nostril and the tips of your index and middle fingers between your eyebrows. Curl your ring and little fingers under, and rest the inside of your ring finger on your left nostril.
- To begin, close your left nostril with your ring finger and exhale fully through your right nostril. Keeping your left nostril closed, inhale fully and slowly through your right nostril. Close your right nostril with your thumb, then release your ring finger to open your left nostril and exhale slowly.
- Pause, then slowly inhale through your left nostril. Close off this nostril with your ring finger. Pause, release your right nostril with your thumb, then exhale slowly and steadily through your right nostril.
- This is one round. Repeat, breathing slowly and mindfully for five minutes.

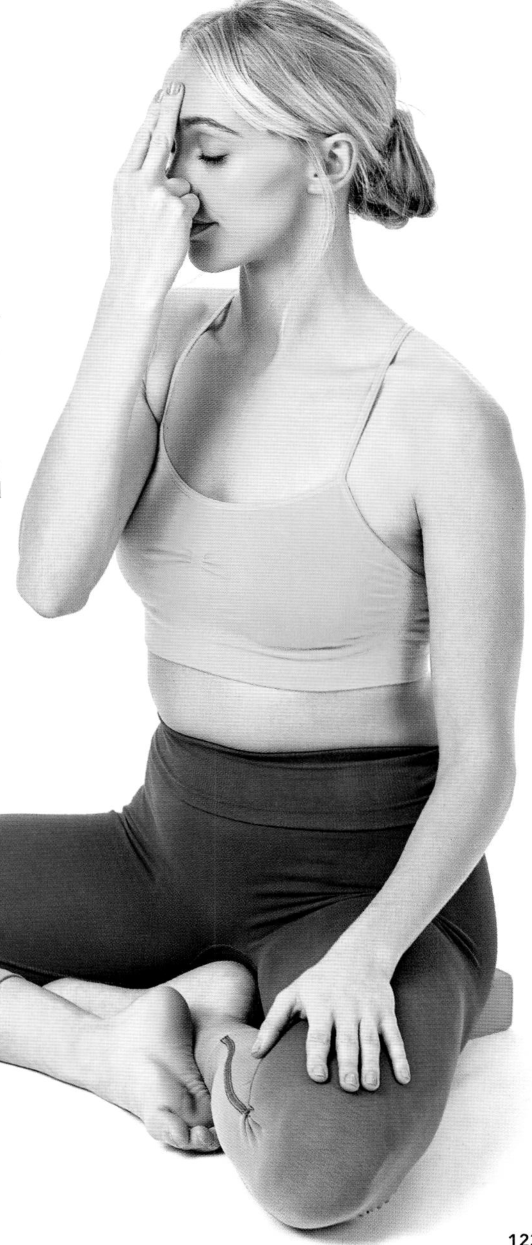

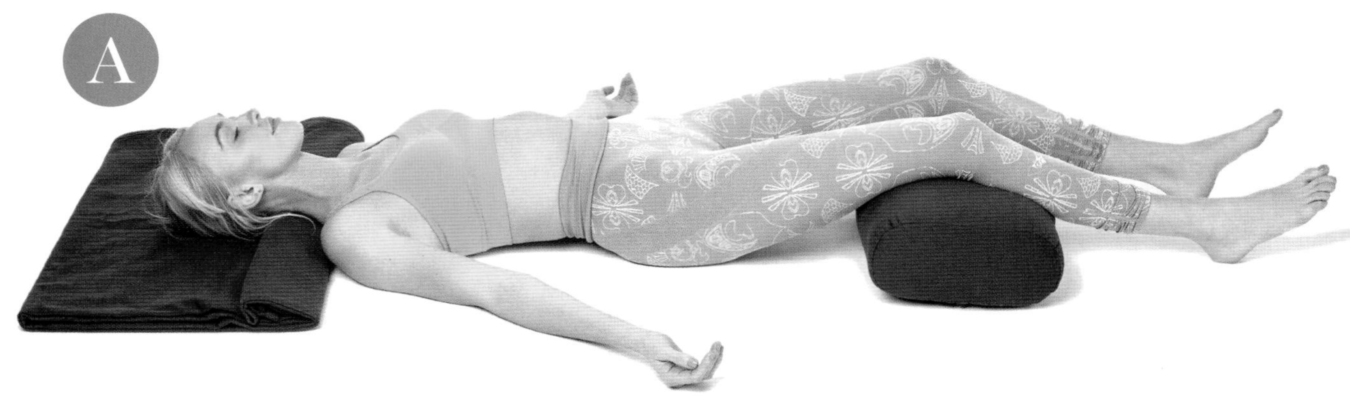

YOGA NIDRA

Often referred to as yogic sleep, Yoga nidra is a state of mind that exists in the space between wakefulness and sleep. It's deeply relaxing and just one hour of Yoga nidra is as restful as four hours' sleep, making it the ideal practice if you have insomnia. What's more, if you do Yoga nidra regularly, you'll soon begin to notice profound changes to your sleeping patterns.

In Yoga nidra you usually listen to a teacher guiding you through a series of instructions, so ask a friend to read you the script below. If this isn't practical, ask them to record it onto your mobile (or you can record it yourself) so you can play it back – though earphones if need be – when you get into bed. The rotation of consciousness (sensing the parts of your body) should be read quite quickly, just giving you enough time to hear and follow the instructions without pausing. Repeat the rotation two or three times, by which time you will probably be asleep!

Lie on your back in Relaxation pose (p67). If comfortable, place a bolster under your knees and a thin blanket under your head, rolled at one end to support your neck (A). If you're lying in bed, turn off the light and rest your head on a pillow, making sure it's not too high as this can create unnecessary tension in your neck.

THE SCRIPT

'Gently close your eyes and become aware of any sounds you can hear outside of your room, acknowledge them, then turn your attention to any sound inside your room. Finally, notice if you can hear the sounds of your own body. Become aware of the sensations where your body is touching the bed, the weight of the duvet, the pressure of the mattress underneath you.

'Begin to count from 20 back down to 1, counting on each exhale. "Exhale, 20, inhale, exhale, 19, inhale, exhale, 18, inhale", and so on... (pause here if making a recording*).

'When you get to "one" pause for a few breaths, then take your awareness from one body part to the next, noticing any sensations you feel there as you repeat the name of the body part in your mind.

'Right side: notice your right thumb, your second finger, middle finger, fourth finger and little finger. Become aware of your right palm, back of your hand, your right wrist, lower arm, elbow upper arm, shoulder, armpit. Notice your right waist, hip, thigh, kneecap, calf muscle, ankle, heel, sole, big toe, second toe, middle toe, fourth toe and little toe.

'Left side: take your attention to your left thumb – repeat as for the right side (if you are recording, read out the instructions as above, changing right for left).

'Back body: now, take your attention to your back. Notice your right shoulder blade, your left shoulder blade, your right buttock, your left buttock, your spine and the whole of your back.

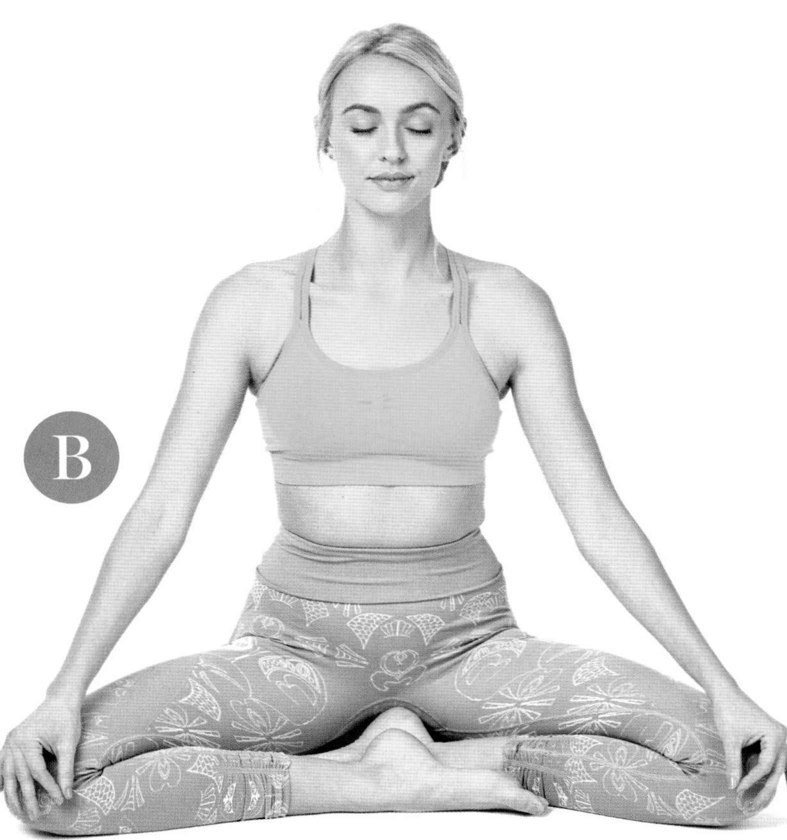

* You can continue breathing in this way yourself as you record, to ensure you begin speaking the rotation of consciousness at the right time.

'Front body: bring your awareness to the top of your head, your forehead, the sides of your head. Notice your right eyebrow, left eyebrow, the space between your eyebrows, your right eyelid, left eyelid, right eye, left eye, right ear, left ear, right cheek and your left cheek. Notice your nose, the tip of your nose, your upper lip, lower lip, chin and throat, your right chest, left chest, middle of your chest, your navel and abdomen.

'Whole body: bring your attention to the whole of your right leg, the whole of your left leg, both legs simultaneously. Notice the whole of your right arm, whole of your left arm, both arms simultaneously. Notice the whole of your back and the back of your legs, the whole of your front and the front of your legs. Be aware of your back and front body simultaneously. Become aware of your head and your body simultaneously. Become aware of your whole body simultaneously.'

SIMPLE MEDITATION ON GOLDEN LIGHT

In the evening, connecting to your breath, becoming still and allowing gentle golden light to surround you is a wonderful way to relax your body and mind, and let go of any negative experiences you may have experienced during the day.

For this practice, place a candle a few feet away from you, so that it is at eye level when you are seating in your meditation position.

Lower the lights in the room, perhaps keeping a small side lamp on, and come into a comfortable seated position (B).

- Gently close your eyes and spend a few moments letting your breath settle and your thoughts recede. Breathe deeply into your lower belly, mid and upper chest, then exhale, releasing the out-breath with a sigh through your open mouth. Repeat two or three times more, feeling the tension in your shoulders melt away. Spend a few more moments breathing into your belly and letting your mind become more and more still. Soften your temples, your jaw and the back of your neck. Let your body become heavy and your sitting bones sink into the mat while maintaining a lift through the crown of your head.
- When you feel ready, gently open your eyes and spend five to 10 minutes gazing at the flame in front of you. Let your eyes be soft. Rather than actively 'look' at the flame, simply allow its gentle light to drift towards you and enter your awareness. Keep breathing gently into your belly and allow yourself to absorb the soft quality of the candlelight. If you notice your mind wandering, gently guide it back to your experience of your body, the movement of your breath, the sensations you feel when gazing at the flame.
- Next, gently close your eyes and take your awareness to the area an arm's distance above the crown of your head. Rest your attention here for a while as you visualise a soft golden light. After a moment or two, imagine the light gently falling and cascading around your body, bathing you in its soft glow. Spend a few minutes allowing the light to expand around your body – in front, to the sides, behind and underneath you – encasing you completely.
- When you feel ready, release the connection, bring your attention to the centre of your forehead, rest here a moment, then take your awareness to your heart. Pause for a moment, bring your hands together in prayer position and gently bow your head.

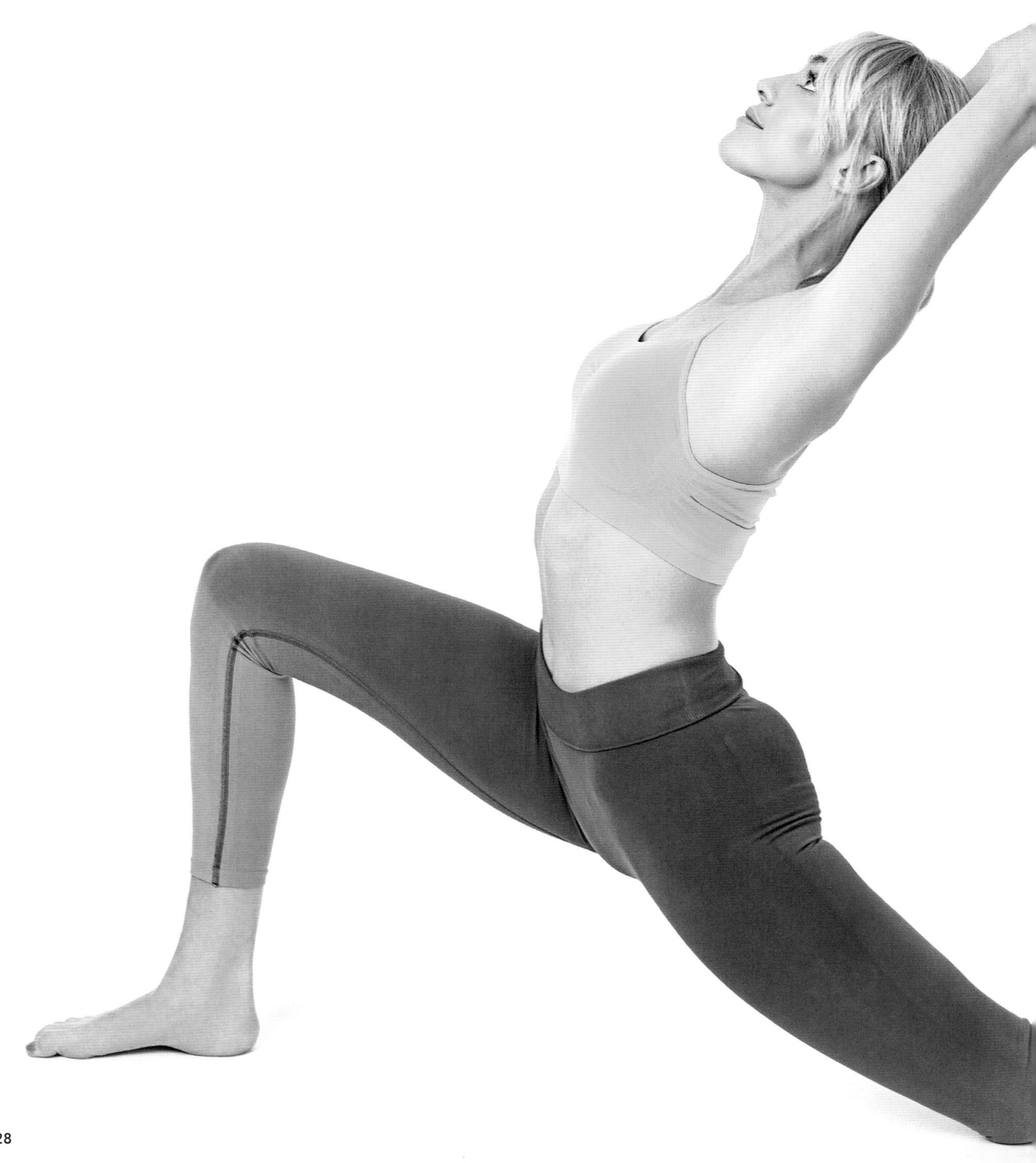

Directory

APPAREL

ACTIVE IN STYLE
activeinstyle.co.uk

ASQUITH
asquithlondon.com

EVERY SECOND COUNTS
everysecondcounts.co.uk

FROMYOGA
fromclothing.com

ILU
ilufitwear.com

LULULEMON
lululemon.co.uk

MADEBYYOGIS
yogaclicks.store

MANDUKA
manduka.com

MANUKA
manukalife.com

NOBALLS
noballs.co.uk

PURE LIME
purelimeshop.com

THE MEDITATION CENTRE
meditationcentre.co.uk

STYLE PB
stylepb.com

SWEATY BETTY
sweatybetty.co.uk

UNDER THE SAME SUN
underthesamesun.se

WELLICIOUS
wellicious.com

EQUIPMENT

GAIAM
gaiam.co.uk

HOLISTIC SILK
holisticsilk.com

MANDUKA
manduka.com

YOGA MATTERS
yogamatters.com

THE YOGA SHOP UK
theyogashop.co.uk

FIND A TEACHER

THE BRITISH WHEEL OF YOGA
bwy.org.uk

YOGA ALLIANCE
yogaalliance.co.uk

TEACHER TRAINING

JUDITH HANSON LASATER
judithhansonlasater.com

SARAH POWERS
sarahpowers.com

SHIVA REA
shivarea.com

TRIYOGA
triyoga.co.uk

YOGA WITH SIMON LOW
simonlow.com

ONLINE YOGA CLASSES

EKART YOGA
ekhartyoga.com

MOVEMENT FOR MODERN LIFE
movementformodernlife.com

GAIA
gaia.com

YOGAGLO
yogaglo.com

YOGAIA
yogaia.com

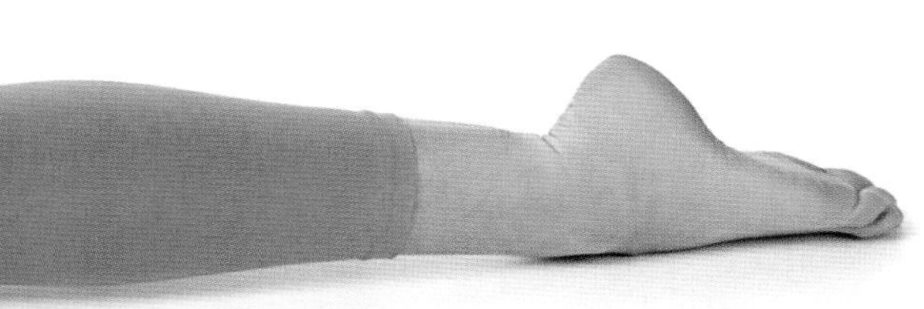

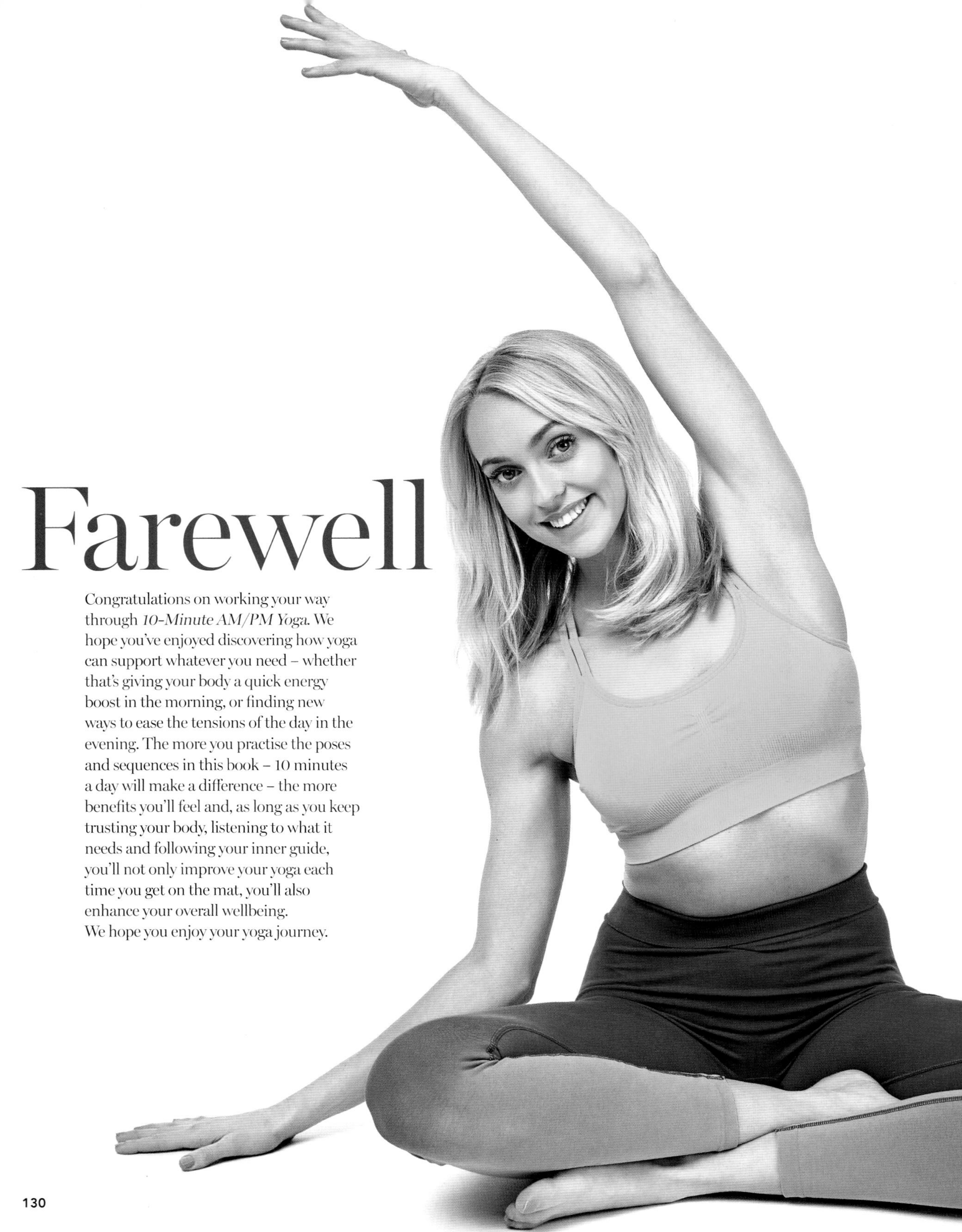

Farewell

Congratulations on working your way through *10-Minute AM/PM Yoga*. We hope you've enjoyed discovering how yoga can support whatever you need – whether that's giving your body a quick energy boost in the morning, or finding new ways to ease the tensions of the day in the evening. The more you practise the poses and sequences in this book – 10 minutes a day will make a difference – the more benefits you'll feel and, as long as you keep trusting your body, listening to what it needs and following your inner guide, you'll not only improve your yoga each time you get on the mat, you'll also enhance your overall wellbeing.
We hope you enjoy your yoga journey.